Rhinoplasty for the Asian Nose

Editor

YONG JU JANG

FACIAL PLASTIC SURGERY CLINICS OF NORTH AMERICA

www.facialplastic.theclinics.com

Consulting Editor
J. REGAN THOMAS

August 2018 • Volume 26 • Number 3

ELSEVIER

1600 John F. Kennedy Boulevard • Suite 1800 • Philadelphia, Pennsylvania, 19103-2899

http://www.theclinics.com

FACIAL PLASTIC SURGERY CLINICS OF NORTH AMERICA Volume 26, Number 3
August 2018 ISSN 1064-7406, ISBN-13: 978-0-323-61386-6

Editor: Jessica McCool
Developmental Editor: Sara Watkins

Facial Plastic Surgery Clinics of North America (ISSN 1064-7406) is published quarterly by Elsevier Inc., 360 Park Avenue South, New York, NY 10010-1710. Months of issue are February, May, August, and November. Business and Editorial Offices: 1600 John F. Kennedy Blvd., Suite 1800, Philadelphia, PA 19103-2899. Periodicals postage paid at New York, NY, and additional mailing offices. Subscription prices are $398.00 per year (US individuals), $628.00 per year (US institutions), $454.00 per year (Canadian individuals), $782.00 per year (Canadian institutions), $535.00 per year (foreign individuals), $782.00 per year (foreign institutions), $100.00 per year (US students), and $255.00 per year (foreign students). Foreign air speed delivery is included in all *Clinics* subscription prices. All prices are subject to change without notice. POSTMASTER: Send address changes to *Facial Plastic Surgery Clinics*, Elsevier Health Sciences Division, Subscription Customer Service, 3251 Riverport Lane, Maryland Heights, MO 63043. **Customer service: 1-800-654-2452 (US and Canada); 1-314-447-8871 (outside US and Canada); Fax: 314-447-8029; E-mail: journalscustomerservice-usa@elsevier.com (for print support); journalsonline support-usa@elsevier.com (for online support).**

Reprints. For copies of 100 or more of articles in this publication, please contact the Commercial Reprints Department, Elsevier Inc., 360 Park Avenue South, New York, NY 10010-1710. Tel.: 212-633-3874; Fax: 212-633-3820; E-mail: reprints@elsevier.com.

Facial Plastic Surgery Clinics of North America is covered in *MEDLINE/PubMed* (*Index Medicus*).

Contributors

CONSULTING EDITOR

J. REGAN THOMAS, MD
Professor, Facial Plastic and Reconstructive
Surgery, Department of Otolaryngology–Head
and Neck Surgery, Northwestern University
Feinberg School of Medicine, Chicago, Illinois,
USA

EDITOR

YONG JU JANG, MD, PhD
Professor, Department of Otolaryngology,
Asan Medical Center, University of Ulsan
College of Medicine, Seoul, Republic of Korea

AUTHORS

JINSOON CHANG, MD, PhD
Department of Otolaryngology–Head and Neck
Surgery, Inje University Seoul Paik Hospital,
Seoul, South Korea

JI YUN CHOI, MD, PhD
Department of Otorhinolaryngology, Chosun
University College of Medicine, Gwangju,
Korea

EUN-SANG DHONG, MD, PhD
Chief, Professor, Department of Plastic and
Reconstructive Surgery, Korea University
College of Medicine, Guro Hospital, Korea
University Medical Center, Seoul, Republic of
Korea

SEUNG-KYU HAN, MD, PhD
Department of Plastic Surgery, Korea
University College of Medicine, Guro Hospital,
Korea University Medical Center, Seoul, South
Korea

NA-HYUN HWANG, MD, MSc
Clinical Instructor, Department of Plastic
and Reconstructive Surgery, Korea University
College of Medicine, Guro Hospital, Korea
University Medical Center, Seoul, Republic of
Korea

SANG MIN HYUN, MD, PhD
Shimmian Rhinoplasty Clinic, Seoul, Republic
of Korea

YONG JU JANG, MD, PhD
Professor, Department of Otolaryngology,
Asan Medical Centre, University of Ulsan
College of Medicine, Seoul, Republic of Korea

SANG GYUN JIN, MD
Shimmian Rhinoplasty Clinic, Seoul, Republic
of Korea

DONG HAK JUNG, MD, PhD
Shimmian Rhinoplasty Clinic, Seoul, Republic
of Korea

JAE-GOO KANG, MD, PhD
Department of Otolaryngology–Head and Neck
Surgery, National Medical Center, Seoul, Korea

CHANG-HOON KIM, MD, PhD
Department of Otorhinolaryngology, The
Airway Mucus Institute, Yonsei University
College of Medicine, Seoul, Korea

IN-SANG KIM, MD
Chief Executive, Doctor Be: Aesthetic Clinic,
Seoul, Korea

SUNG HEE KIM, MD
Department of Otolaryngology, National
Medical Centre, Seoul, Republic of Korea

KYUNG WON KWON, MD
Department of Otolaryngology–Head and Neck
Surgery, National Medical Center, Seoul, Korea

HYOUNG JIN MOON, MD
Director, Beup Aesthetic Plastic Surgery Clinic,
Seoul, Republic of Korea

KYUNG-CHUL MOON, MD, PhD
Department of Plastic Surgery, Korea
University College of Medicine, Guro Hospital,
Korea University Medical Center, Seoul, South
Korea

SANG CHUL PARK, MD
Department of Otorhinolaryngology, Yonsei
University College of Medicine, Seoul, Korea

MAN-KOON SUH, MD
Director, JW Plastic Surgery Center, Seoul,
Republic of Korea

TAE-BIN WON, MD, PhD
Associate Professor, Department of
Otorhinolaryngology–Head and Neck Surgery,
Seoul National University Hospital, Seoul,
Republic of Korea

EDUARDO C. YAP, MD, FPSO-HNS
Consultant, Section of Facial Plastic Surgery,
Belo Medical Group, Manila, Philippines

Contents

Preface: Truly Asian Rhinoplasty ix

Yong Ju Jang

Surgical Anatomy of the Asian Nose 259

Kyung-Chul Moon and Seung-Kyu Han

Rhinoplasty for Asian noses is markedly different from that for white noses. As rhinoplasty becomes increasingly popular among Asian people, it is important that the rhinoplasty surgeons master relevant anatomy and become skilled in required techniques to serve this segment of population. In this article, distinct characteristics of Asian noses are briefly described. Noses in the Asian population exhibit broad phenotypic variations. There is no typical Asian nose. Therefore, the terms of Asian noses in this article are confined to noses of people from East Asia (eg, Korea, Japan, and China).

Hybrid Approach for Asian Rhinoplasty: Open Approach Without Transcolumellar Incision 269

Jae-Goo Kang, Kyung Won Kwon, and Jinsoon Chang

The hybrid approach delivers unlimited exposure and technical access, enabling all the procedures of the open approach. In addition, the hybrid approach is flexible in its extent of "dissection/exposure." It can be more of a classic endonasal or limited access approach in some cases or open structural rhinoplasty and reconstruction in others. The benefits of the nonopen approach deserve equal attention among Asian rhinoplasty surgeons and residents-in-training courses. The difference is not merely that it spares an incision, it is an opportunity to fine-tune minor millimeters of changes in every step of rhinoplasty, a real and significant benefit.

Augmentation Rhinoplasty Using Silicone Implants 285

In-Sang Kim

Augmentation rhinoplasty is one of the most common aesthetic procedures in Asian countries, with silicone implant being the most widely used material. Despite potential advantages, use of alloplastic materials in rhinoplasty is often discouraged in Western countries because of concern for possible risk of infection and extrusion of the implant. The collective experience of long-term favorable outcomes in Asia makes the silicone augmentation rhinoplasty a common procedure. Complication rates for silicone implants vary significantly, depending on surgeon experience, surgical technique, and implant design. Silicone implants can be safely used for nasal dorsal augmentation if precautions are taken.

Dorsal Augmentation Using Autogenous Tissues 295

Man-Koon Suh

Autogenous materials used for Asian dorsal augmentation are temporal fascia, dermofat, solid block type of costal cartilage, and diced cartilage. The temporal fascia is used for radix augmentation or correction of minor focal depression. Dermofat, solid block costal cartilage, and diced cartilage are recommended for major dorsal augmentation. The vertically oriented folded dermal graft curtails use of the fat component. Diced cartilage wrapped in temporal fascia exhibits a lower resorption rate and may easily fit into the contour of the dorsum. This graft is thought to have low predictability of final height, as opposed to that of block cartilage.

Homologous Tissue for Dorsal Augmentation   311

Chang-Hoon Kim and Sang Chul Park

Homologous graft materials for dorsal augmentation are safe and biocompatible with a low risk of complications. Acellular dermal matrix (ADM) provides natural appearance of the nose and long-term structural integrity without extrusion, showing favorable augmentation results. Tutoplast-processed fascia lata (TPFL) is soft and easy to manipulate, providing a smooth postoperative contour of the nasal dorsum with low risk of infection or extrusion. ADM and TPFL carry low risk of major complications, such as infection, foreign body reaction, and graft extrusion. ADM and TPFL are suitable graft materials that deliver proper dorsal augmentation and patient satisfaction in primary and revision rhinoplasty.

Injection Rhinoplasty Using Filler   323

Hyoung Jin Moon

Rhinoplasty is a commonly performed cosmetic surgery in Asia. Rhinoplasty using filler is preferred because it has fewer side effects and a shorter down time. The part of external nose between the skin and bone or cartilages consists of 4 layers. To prevent vascular compromise, the injection should be into the deep fatty layer, preventing embolization. The filler is usually injected in the order of radix, rhinion, tip, and the supratip area. To minimize asymmetry, the surgeon should always mark the midline on the nasal bridge and perform the procedure without deviating from it.

Septal Extension Graft in Asian Rhinoplasty   331

Na-Hyun Hwang and Eun-Sang Dhong

 Video content accompanies this article at http://www.facialplastic.theclinics.com.

A septal extension graft (SEG) can control nasal tip projection, shape, and rotation. SEG and dorsal alloplastic implants have predominated in Asian rhinoplasty, leading to iatrogenic complications such as a foreshortened nose and destruction of the remaining septum. The lower nasal two-thirds can be enhanced anteriorly and caudally using the septal L-strut extension graft in Asians with relatively small noses. The septal L-strut extension graft is indicated in primary cases in which the bony dorsum is acceptable but the cartilaginous dorsum is relatively hypoplastic and in secondary cases with an iatrogenic short-nose deformity due to alloplastic implants.

Tip Grafting for the Asian Nose   343

Yong Ju Jang and Sung Hee Kim

 Video content accompanies this article at http://www.facialplastic.theclinics.com.

Tip surgery during rhinoplasty is particularly difficult in Asians. Tip grafting is the best approach. Conchal cartilage with perichondrium and costal cartilage are powerful grafting materials. The most important grafting techniques are tip-onlay grafting, shield grafting, and multilayer tip grafting. Tip-onlay grafts are useful for dorsal convexity. Shield grafts require sufficient support to prevent bending. Multilayer tip grafts (usually 2 layers) are versatile. Asians vary in cartilage configuration, skin thickness, and aesthetic desires: tip-grafting strategies must be tailored to meet the aesthetic goals of individuals. Tip-grafting complications (eg, visible graft contour and infection) are not uncommon and should be considered.

Hump Nose Correction in Asians   357

Tae-Bin Won

 Video content accompanies this article at http://www.facialplastic.theclinics.com.

Nasal hump surgery is frequently regarded as a reduction surgery in most Western rhinoplasty textbooks and referred to as reduction rhinoplasty. Most Asian hump noses have a small hump frequently associated with a low nasal dorsum and under-projection of the nasal tip. Correcting a hump nose in Asians has distinct differences in concept and technique. A small hump and additional need for augmentation of the dorsum and the tip often minimizes the amount of hump removal or obviates resection itself. Characteristics of the Asian hump nose with emphasis on surgical techniques commonly used to obtain reliable results are presented.

Alar Base Reduction and Alar-Columellar Relationship   367

Ji Yun Choi

Nasal base modification can improve nostril shape and orientation, reduce alar flaring, improve nasal base width, correct nasal hooding, improve symmetry, and create overall facial harmony. For the correction of alar rim deformities, careful examination, consultation, and analysis and consideration of the condition of the skin are essential. Understanding the ala and surrounding tissue, supporting the lower lateral cartilage, and selecting the proper technique produce functionally and aesthetically good results.

Correction of Short Nose   377

Dong Hak Jung, Sang Gyun Jin, and Sang Min Hyun

To correct an Asian short nose with a low dorsum, short columella, and poorly defined nose tip, augmentation rhinoplasty has been popularized. A simple augmentation no longer is considered an efficient rhinoplasty approach for Asians aesthetically; most surgeons simultaneously perform nasal elongation and augmentation during rhinoplasty. To extend the nose length successfully, important factors are cartilages, mucosal and skin conditions, and presence and degree of fibrotic changes. In addition, surgeons should consider preoperatively how much should be extended from an aesthetics perspective. This article introduces the current practice of surgical correction of the short nose in Asians.

Rhinoplasty for South East Asian Nose   389

Eduardo C. Yap

The South East Asian nose is usually small with voluminous thick skin, low dorsum, wide and hanging ala, bulbous tip, and retracted premaxilla. The surgical approach of rhinoplasty for these types of noses includes the following: dorsal augmentation, counterrotation and projection of the tip, and correction of hanging ala and alar flare/base. A usual ideal rhinoplasty outcome of a South East Asian nose should be a nose that fits the face with good function and has all the aesthetic landmarks achieved: natural looking dorsum, supratip break, tip, subtip break, columellar show, good alar-columellar relationship, improved premaxilla, improved nostril, and improved alar flare.

FACIAL PLASTIC SURGERY CLINICS OF NORTH AMERICA

FORTHCOMING ISSUES

November 2018
Current Utilization of Biologicals
Greg Keller, *Editor*

February 2019
Skin Cancer Surgery
Jeffrey S. Moyer, *Editor*

May 2019
Facial Gender Affirmation Surgery
Michael T. Somenek, *Editor*

RECENT ISSUES

May 2018
Controversies in Facial Plastic Surgery
Fred G. Fedok and Robert M. Kellman, *Editors*

February 2018
Cosmetic and Reconstructive Surgery of Congenital Ear Deformities
Scott Stephan, *Editor*

November 2017
Trauma in Facial Plastic Surgery
Kris S. Moe, *Editor*

RELATED INTEREST

Hand Clinics, August 2017 (Vol. 33, No. 3)
Hand Surgery in Asia and Europe
Jin Bo Tang and Grey Giddins, *Editors*
Available at: http://www.hand.theclinics.com/

THE CLINICS ARE AVAILABLE ONLINE!
Access your subscription at:
www.theclinics.com

Preface
Truly Asian Rhinoplasty

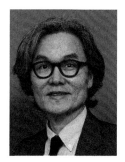

Yong Ju Jang, MD, PhD
Editor

It is a well-recognized fact that there is a distinctive quality to Asian Rhinoplasty when compared with rhinoplasty for patients from other regions. For Asian patients, especially from East and Southeast Asia, the relatively smaller sized noses have made simple augmentation of the nose using alloplastic implant stand in for the term "Rhinoplasty." However, with growing understanding of the diverse anatomical features of Asian noses and an increased sophistication in patients' aesthetic demands, Asian surgeons came to realize that "Asian Rhinoplasty" can be far more complex. This revelatory insight into Asian rhinoplasty has helped Asian surgeons rapidly expand the variety of rhinoplasty techniques employed in our everyday practice for the past 25 years.

At the same time, the world is witnessing both an increase in migration of Asian people to all parts of the world and an increase in interracial marriage. Hence, rhinoplasty for the Asian nose is no longer exclusive to Asian surgeons. To cope with the growing demand for learning about Asian rhinoplasty, publications on Asian rhinoplasty are correspondingly increasing.

In this era of burgeoning interest in Asian rhinoplasty, it was a great pleasure and honor for me to take responsibility of editing an issue about Asian rhinoplasty, which will be a special issue dedicated solely to Asian Rhinoplasty, of the esteemed *Facial Plastic Surgery Clinics of North America*.

In preparation for this issue, I thought about a few things: the content should be comprehensive;

authors should be Asia-based experts who are keen to teach and have distinct areas of interest; and the content should be up-to-date. With those considerations in mind, I invited 10 eminent surgeons from Korea, and 1 surgeon from the Philippines. I am deeply grateful to the invited authors for the phenomenal effort that they have put into preparing their outstanding articles. The issue covers anatomy, surgical approach, dorsal augmentation using silicone, augmentation using homologous tissue, injection rhinoplasty, septal extension grafting, nasal tip grafting, hump nose correction, alar base reduction and alar-columellar relationship, correction of short nose, and rhinoplasty for the Southeast Asian nose. All articles provide clear insight into various aspects of Asian rhinoplasty techniques that can only be generated by genuine masters of each field. I believe that this special issue will enrich the readers' armamentarium for Asian rhinoplasty. It will also contribute greatly to improving rhinoplasty outcome for patients who have similar anatomical features with Asian noses and for revision cases of other ethnicities that need structural grafting and augmentation.

One thing I am not happy with my editing is that I could not feature surgeons from China, Taiwan, and Japan as contributors. However, I am confident that the content provided in this special issue will represent contemporary rhinoplasty practice in East Asia. In addition, due to constraints in length, I feel sorry for not being

Facial Plast Surg Clin N Am 26 (2018) ix–x
https://doi.org/10.1016/j.fsc.2018.03.013
1064-7406/18/© 2018 Published by Elsevier Inc.

facialplastic.theclinics.com

able to include other important topics, such as deviated nose, septal surgery, and reconstructive surgery.

Last, I do hope this collective endeavor of the contributing authors can help the readers get a better understanding of rhinoplasty for Asian noses. Ideally, this better understanding can translate into better surgical outcomes and, ultimately, actualized into better patient care.

Yong Ju Jang, MD, PhD
Department of Otolaryngology
Asan Medical Center
University of Ulsan College of Medicine
88 Olympic-ro 43-gil, Songpa-gu
Seoul 05505, Republic of Korea

E-mail address:
jangyj@amc.seoul.kr

Surgical Anatomy of the Asian Nose

Kyung-Chul Moon, MD, PhD, Seung-Kyu Han, MD, PhD*

KEYWORDS

• Asian nose • Nose anatomy • Nostril shape

KEY POINTS

- Dilator naris and depressor septi nasi muscles are well developed in most Asians who have horizontally oriented nostrils.
- Lateral crus shape of the alar cartilage and length of the footplate segment of the medial crus influence the shape of nostril.
- Characteristics of tip supporting structures contributes to the nasal tip of Asians appearing broad and unprojected with wide bases.

Rhinoplasty for Asian noses is markedly different from that for white noses. As rhinoplasty becomes increasingly popular among Asian people, it is important that the rhinoplasty surgeons master relevant anatomy and become skilled in required techniques to serve this segment of population.

In this article, distinct characteristics of Asian noses are briefly described. We emphasize two points. First, subjects that have been dealt with elsewhere (eg, general anatomy of the nose) were omitted from this article. Thus, trainees in rhinoplasty surgery might need to obtain information for these neglected subjects from elsewhere. Second, noses in the Asia population exhibit broad phenotypic variations. There is no typical Asian nose. Therefore, the terms of Asian noses in this article are confined to noses of people from East Asian (eg, Korea, Japan, and China).

This article provides a rational basis for understanding the anatomy of Asian noses and advancing surgical skills for Asian rhinoplasty.

EXTERNAL NOSE

Asian noses are generally described as having bulbous tip, short columella, flared nostril shape, wide alar base, acute nasolabial angle (NLA), and low dorsum.[1] The average nasal length/dorsal height/radix height ratio of the nose in white people has been shown to be 2:1:0.75.[2] However, in Asian people it is 2:0.61:0.28.[3]

The nasal dorsum and the tip are the most commonly addressed structures in Asian rhinoplasty. Dorsal nasal augmentation and nasal tip refinement are the most important parts in Asian rhinoplasty. Changes in morphology of these two structures can influence nasofrontal angle (NFA) and NLA of the face. Emphasizing enhancement of natural beauty and knowledge of the two angles are essential elements in Asian rhinoplasty. Attaining ideal NFA and NLA is the key to have successful and aesthetically pleasing results in Asian rhinoplasty.

In performing augmentation rhinoplasty using an implant, precise positioning of the cephalic end of a nasal implant is important. Generally, men tend to prefer higher radix than women.[4,5] Traditional dorsal nasal augmentation predisposes to radix elevation. In some cases, radix elevation might efface or eliminate the radix, resulting in elevated radix deformity.[6] Yu and Jang[7] have reported

Disclosure: K.-C. Moon and S.-K. Han have nothing to disclose.
Department of Plastic Surgery, Korea University College of Medicine, Korea University Guro Hospital, 148 Guro-Dong, Guro-Ku, Seoul 152-703, South Korea
* Corresponding author.
E-mail address: pshan@kumc.or.kr

Facial Plast Surg Clin N Am 26 (2018) 259–268
https://doi.org/10.1016/j.fsc.2018.03.001

that Asians who undergo rhinoplasty prefer an NFA of 138°.

Defining NLA as the angle between the inferior border of the nose on lateral view and the labial surface of the upper lip,[8–10] ideal NLA has been classically reported to be 95° to 100° in men and 103° to 108° in women.[10–12] Sinno and colleagues[13] have reported that there is no clear statistically significant preference for the most aesthetic NLA between white persons and Asians. However, in Asian noses, the tip rotates caudally with an acute NLA ranging from 70° to 80°.[14]

In terms of nasal bridge length (the distance between the sellion and pronasale) and cartilaginous nasal bridge length (the distance between the rhinion and pronasale), they are significantly shorter in Asians than those in white persons.[15]

SKIN AND SUBCUTANEOUS TISSUE

Characteristics of the skin and subcutaneous layer of Asian noses are often described as being variable in thickness and oiliness. According to research using computed tomography scans of Korean noses, the mean nasal skin thickness is 3.3 mm at the nasion, 2.4 mm at the rhinion, 2.9 mm for the nasal tip, and 2.3 mm for the columella. In that study, thick skin at nasal tip and columella is associated with poorer surgical outcomes, suggesting that regional skin thickness is an important prognostic factor for tip surgery success.[16]

Like white persons, the subcutaneous layer in Asian noses is made up of three layers: (1) superficial fatty layer, (2) nasal superficial muscular aponeurotic system (SMAS) layer, and (3) deep fatty layer (**Fig. 1**).[17] Although nasal SMAS of the upper nose is well defined and easily dissected, SMAS is anchored more securely in the lower nose and it is not well-defined yet. Major nerves and vessels run within the deep fatty layer. Tansatit and colleagues[18] have reported that the thickness of the soft tissue from the skin to the frontal bone at the glabella in Asian noses is 7.2 ± 2.1 mm and it is narrowed down to 3.1 ± 1.8 mm at the radix and over the nasal bone. Thickness of the tissue is increased to 5.7 ± 3.4 mm above the lateral and major alar cartilages.

The soft tissue covering the lower one-third of the nose is important in nasal tip plasty. The skin of the lower third of the nose is thicker and oilier than that of the upper part. The subcutaneous layer is not distinct. Therefore, it is difficult to discriminate it from the skin and muscle layers. The anatomy of this area differs according to alar lobule or nostril shape. Depending on the prominence and roundness of alar lobules, they are classified as horizontal (flaring) or vertical (straight).

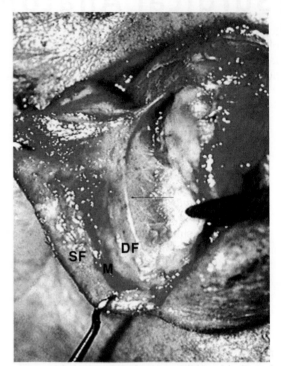

Fig. 1. Subcutaneous layers of the nose. DF, deep fatty layer; M, nasal SMAS layer; SF, superficial fatty layer. External nasal nerve running within the deep fatty layer (*arrow*).

Based on data from dissections of 20 fresh cadavers, the thickness of the skin in alar lobule of Asian noses is between 1.25 mm and 2.75 mm.[17] External skin thickness of the lateral alar lobule tends to differ according to nostril shape, with the skin of the horizontal (flaring)-type being thicker than that of the vertical (straight)-type.

MUSCLES OF THE EXTERNAL NOSE

The distinct shape of Asian noses is affected by the pull of nasal muscles surrounding the external nose. External nasal muscles include the dilator naris anterior and posterior, transverse nasalis, levator labii superioris alaque nasi, and depressor septi nasi muscles. They are identified by careful subcutaneous dissection. The compressor narium minor is rarely seen grossly. Sometimes it is identified microscopically.[17,19,20]

There are significant differences in the characteristics of some nasal muscles with respect to nostril shape. In general, nasal muscles of alar lobules in nostrils with a horizontal shape are more developed compared with those with vertical shape. They have an obtuse angle formed by the long axis of the nostril, rather than acute angles of nostrils with vertical shape. These differences are the focus of this article.[17,19,20]

The dilator naris anterior is the primary dilator of the nose, widening the ala as it contracts. This muscle might be involved in enlarging nostrils and maintaining the laterally extruding alae. The dilator naris anterior muscle is well developed in nostrils with horizontal shape, but poorly developed in vertically oriented nostrils. In horizontal-type nostrils, this muscle and its origin from the upper lateral cartilage with insertion into the caudal margin of the lateral crus and alar lobule skin is easily identified. Conversely, identification of the dilator naris anterior in nostrils with vertical-type is difficult. In addition, the muscle layer volume of horizontally oriented nostrils is significantly larger than that of vertically oriented nostrils (**Fig. 2**).[17,19,20]

The function of the dilator naris posterior or the alar nasalis is to draw ala and the posterior part of the columella downward, widening the nasal aperture and elongating the nose. This muscle is also involved in enlarging nostrils and maintaining the laterally extruding alae. Unlike vertically oriented nostrils where the insertion of the dilator naris posterior is limited to the alar base only, the insertion of the dilator naris posterior in horizontally oriented nostrils is extended to the alar lobule and the alar base.[17,19,20] The muscle layer of horizontally oriented nostrils is also significantly thicker than that of vertically oriented nostrils. By cutting and thereby weakening the well-developed alar nasalis muscles, their function in maintaining the shape of the ala is reduced, thus lessening rounding and flaring.[21]

The depressor septi nasi muscle is inserted into the columella, the membranous septum, and the base of the medial crura of the lower lateral cartilage. This muscle functions by drawing down the

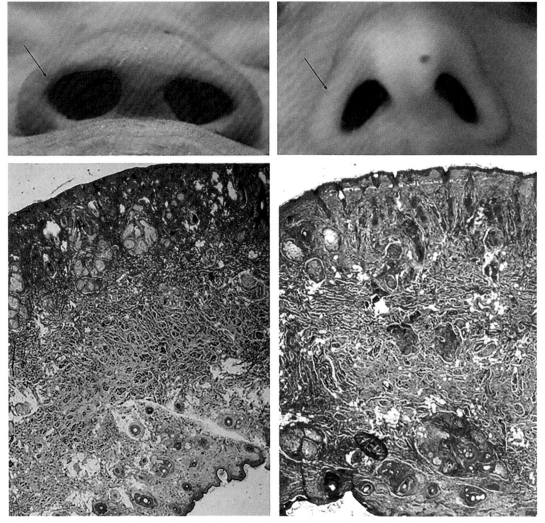

Fig. 2. Histology of the alar lobule midpoint showing dilator naris anterior muscles (Masson trichrome stain, original magnification x40). Horizontal-type nostrils (*left*) showing more muscle volume than vertical-types (*right*).

columella, the tip of the nose, and the dorsal border of the nostril. Although the depressor septi nasi muscle is associated with nasal tip drooping, it also affects nostril shape. In horizontal-type nostrils, the depressor septi nasi muscle is attached to the footplate of the medial crus, extending to the columellar segment, the columellar and vestibular skin, and the membranous septum. However, in vertically oriented nostrils, the attachment of the depressor septi nasi muscle is either confined to the footplate of the medial crus or the muscle does not reach the footplate at all. Instead, it terminates toward the skin of the columellar base (**Fig. 3**).[17,19,20]

The transverse nasalis elongates the nose and compresses the vestibule, producing a pinched or flattened nose. The characteristics of transverse nasalis are not significantly different according to nostril shape. In either nostril type, this muscle does not extend toward the alar lobule. Muscle width is not significantly different between the two nostril types.[17,19,20]

The levator labii superioris alaque nasi has the same characteristics for both nostril types. All of its muscle fibers are inserted into the nasolabial fold and muscles of the upper lip without attaching to the alar lobule.[17,19,20]

The compressor narium minor is a small muscle whose presence has been inconsistently reported. Grossly, the compressior narium minor is not apparent in most Asian noses. Microscopically, the compressior narium minor muscle layer has been identified at the nostril apex in about 10% of noses. This muscle does not seem to affect the shape of nostril.

The anomalous nasi muscle has been reported to exist between the transverse nasalis muscle and the levator labii superioris alaque nasi muscle

in white noses. However, it is not identifiable in most Asian noses.[17,19,20]

NASAL TIP SUPPORTING STRUCTURES

It is generally agreed that important components of nasal tip support in white noses include the attachment between upper and lower lateral cartilages, the attachment between lateral crus of the lower lateral cartilage and the pyriform aperture, the attachment between paired domes of lower lateral cartilages, the medial crural attachment of the lower lateral cartilage to the caudal septum, and Pitanguy dermocartilaginous ligament (**Fig. 4**).[22–24] However, there is no universally agreed consensus for terms of and definitions of these structures. The structure between the upper and lower lateral cartilages has been described as fibrous tissue or connection, intercartilaginous ligament, ligament-like arrangement, or connective tissue. The structure between the lateral crus and the pyriform aperture has been described as definite fibrous attachment or ligamentous fibrous tissue. The structure between paired domes of the lower lateral cartilages has been described as interdomal ligament, suspensory ligament, or dense irregularly interwoven connective tissue. The structure between the medial crus and the caudal septum has been described as loose connection, membranous attachment, or ligamentous attachment. In some cases, it is not described as an attachment at all.

Nasal tip supporting structures play an important role in nasal tip plasty. In fact, these supporting elements of the nasal tip are often severed during the course of routine rhinoplasty by maneuvers, such as complete transfixion incisions, intercartilaginous incisions, reduction of the septal angle, and incising or excising cuts into the lower

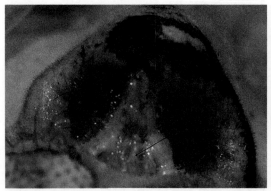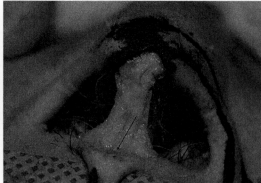

Fig. 3. The depressor septi nasi of a horizontal-type nostril (*left*) attaches to the medial crus, vestibular skin, and columellar skin (*arrows*). The depressor septi nasi of a vertical-type nostril (*right*). The end of the depressor septi nasi in a vertical-type nostril does not reach the footplate of the medial crura and columellar skin (*arrow*).

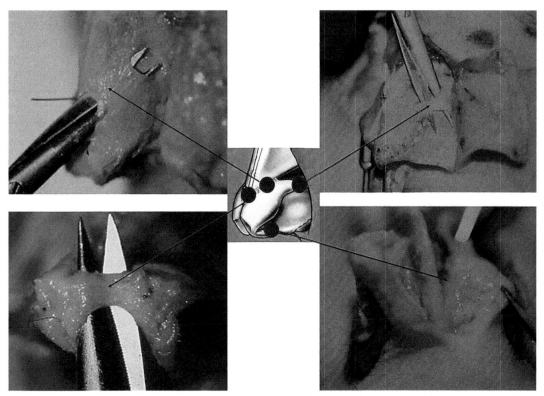

Fig. 4. Nasal tip supporting structures include the attachment between the upper and lower lateral cartilages (*above, left*), the attachment between the lateral crus of the lower lateral cartilage and the pyriform aperture (*above, right*), the attachment between the paired domes of the lower lateral cartilages (*below, left*), and the medial crural attachment of the lower lateral cartilage to the caudal septum (*below, right*). Pitanguy dermocartilaginous ligament is not shown.

lateral cartilage. Thus, a clear understanding of these structures is essential to rhinoplasty surgeons. Lee and colleagues[25] have attempted to exactly define supporting structures of the nasal tip by microscopic investigation in parallel with macroscopic findings specifically for Asian noses whose structural aspects are different from those of white noses.

In Asian noses, the dense fibrous tissue connecting the upper lateral cartilage and the lateral crus is grossly observed. Between the two cartilages, abundant amounts of dense collagen fibers are regularly arranged in one direction. However, a small amount of amorphous ground substance is observed. From histologic point of view, this finding corresponds to dense regular connective tissue. Specifically, the connection is strongly attached to both cartilages, consistent with the definition of a ligament.[22,23]

With respect to the structure between the lateral crus and the pyriform aperture, sesamoid cartilages and dense fibrous tissue are grossly observed. Microscopic examination of this area reveals the existence of an abundant amount of

collagen fibers and muscle fibers. These collagen fibers have some inconsistency, showing both regular and irregular arrangements. This area is also made of small amounts of elastic fibers, cells, and amorphous ground substances. From a histologic point of view, this structure could be fibromuscular tissue.[22,23]

Macroscopic examination for Asian noses reveals that loose tissue fills the area between paired domes of the lower lateral cartilages. Microscopic examination shows that the tissue in this place is composed of abundant amorphous ground substances. In addition, small amounts of collagen and elastic fibers are scattered throughout the section. Based on its histologic aspects, this might be loose connective tissue.[22,23]

For the attachment between the medial crus and the caudal septum, no remarkable supporting structure is identifiable in Asian noses.[22,23]

The dermocartilaginous ligament of the nose is a narrow, central, fibrous, and white structure in the center of the nasal dorsum, and was first described by Pitanguy and coworkers.[26] This structure is believed to unite the dermis of the upper third of the nose to the junction of the medial crura, reaching down to the subseptum. Therefore, the dermocartilaginous ligament can influence the equilibrium of dorsum-tip relationship. In Asian noses, a white dense fibrous band runs vertically between the transverse nasalis muscle and the columellar base. This structure originates from the deep layer of the transverse nasalis muscle and terminates at the caudal edge of the septal cartilage. In some patients (19%), the insertion extends to the orbicularis oris (**Fig. 5**). Histologically, this structure is composed of dense and irregularly arranged connective tissue (ie, a "fascia"). Therefore, the dermocartilaginous ligament in Asian people might be renamed median musculocartilaginous fascia.[24]

With respect to the nasal tip supporting structures, there are two significant characteristics of Asian noses. First, loose connective tissue exists only between paired domes of the lower lateral cartilages, contributing to longer distance between alar domes. Second, a significant supporting structure is not present at the attachment between the medial crus of the lower lateral

cartilage and the caudal septum. Therefore, the footplate segment of the medial crus is longer than the columellar segment in typical Asian noses. These two characteristics contribute to the nasal tip of Asians appearing broad and unprojected with a wide base.[22,23]

CARTILAGES

The alar cartilage consists of lateral, middle, and medial crura. The size and strength of paired alar cartilages are among main factors that determine the shape of the nasal tip. Considering the vast array of anatomic differences between white and Asian nasal configurations, surgical approach should also be distinctively different.

Alar cartilages in Asians are thin and weak, affording little support to the overlaying thick skin and fibrofatty unit. Considering that manipulation of alar cartilages has increased its popularity in Asian rhinoplasty, the first step should be proper and appropriate manipulation of the tripod formed by the two lateral crura and the medial crura.

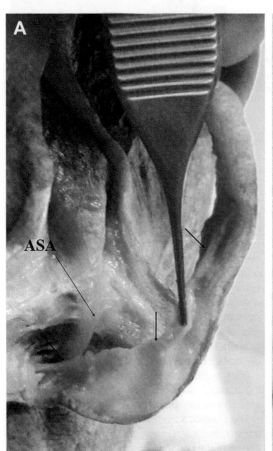
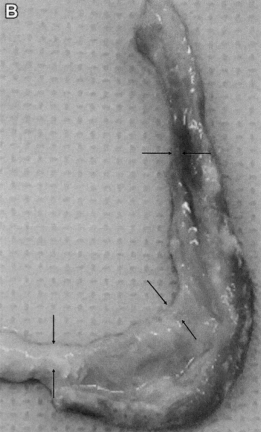

Fig. 5. (*A, B*) The dermocartilaginous ligament (*arrows*) inserts into the orbicularis oris muscle tissue and the septal cartilage (the septal cartilage insertion portion is divided). ASA, anterior septal angle.

In the study by Zelnik and Gingrass,[27] the mean length and width of lateral crus in white persons are 22 mm and 11 mm, respectively. However, Ofodile and James[28] have performed similar studies on black male cadavers and found that the mean length and width are 18 mm and 12 mm, respectively. In Asians, the average length, width, and thickness of lateral crus are 18 mm, 10 mm, and 5 mm, respectively. The medial, middle, and lateral distance of lateral crus from nostril rim are 5.8 mm, 6.9 mm, and 11.8 mm, respectively. Morphologic types of lateral crura are classified into concave, convex, concave-convex, convex-concave, and flat. Shapes of lateral crura in Asians are dissimilar compared with those in white or black persons. The most common shape of the Asian nose is concave. It has been found in 40% of male patients and 50% of female patients. However, the convex-concave shape, which is the most common one in other races, has been found in 30% of white persons and 50% of black persons. Comparison between the right crus and the left crus has indicated that 7% of patients have asymmetric configuration of the lateral crura.[29]

The concept of a middle crus was first introduced by Sheen and Sheen in 1987.[30] In white noses, the middle crus is made of lobular segment and domal segment. In Asian noses, it is almost impossible to divide the middle crus into lobular and domal segments because the middle crural configuration is typically flat. The length of middle crus is measured from the point of divergence of the medial crura to the dome. Its average length in Asian noses is 4.9 mm (**Fig. 6**).[29]

The length of the medial crus is measured individually into columellar segment and footplate segment from the point of divergence. Guyuron[31] has conducted prospective measurements for footplate segments and reported that the average length is 5.8 mm (range, 4–7.5 mm). In Asian noses, average lengths of the columellar segment and footplate segment are 8.7 mm and 6.9 mm, respectively (**Fig. 7**). Their average width and thickness are 4.3 mm and 0.6 mm, respectively. This suggests that a surgeon can use a longer and more posteriorly angulated footplate segment for Asian noses. This is one of the most important differences between Asian and white noses and it might recreate lower vault of the nose for Asians more effectively than that for white persons. Morphologic types of the medial crura are usually classified as straight, simple flared, and complex flared. Straight-type is the most common, and only 5% of Asian patients have asymmetric shape of medial crura.[29]

Septal cartilage may be the most commonly used cartilage for rhinoplasty in white persons because it lies within the operation field without needing additional donor. In addition, the flat nature and hardness of the septal cartilage make it an optimal choice for rhinoplasty.[32] However, the use of septal cartilage is not always available in Asian rhinoplasty because the amount of harvested septal cartilage is commonly not enough for cartilage grafting procedures. Kim and colleagues[33] have measured the size of harvested septal cartilage intraoperatively with preservation of L struts 10 mm wide. The mean caudal length of the harvested septal cartilage is 15.1 mm and the mean dorsal length is 18.2 mm. Therefore, the size and quantity of harvestable septal cartilage may be inadequate for complex rhinoplasty procedures, increasing the need of harvesting grafts from other sites. Kim and colleagues[15] have measured areas of the septal cartilage using computed tomography scanning. In white persons, areas of the septal cartilage in men and

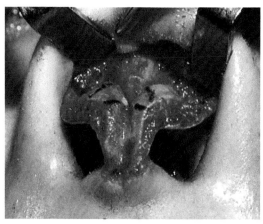

Fig. 6. Shape of the flat middle crura. This structure is identifiable in most Asian noses.

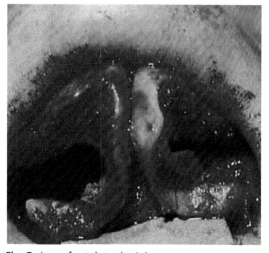

Fig. 7. Long footplates in Asian noses.

women are 998 and 861 mm^2, respectively. In Asians, those in men and women are 962 and 750 mm^2, respectively. Therefore, septal cartilage is significantly larger in white females than that in Asian females. However, there is no significant difference between white males and Asian males.

STRUCTURES DETERMINING NOSTRIL SHAPE OF ASIAN NOSES

Aesthetically acceptable nostril is described as teardrop-shaped, with a long axis from its base to the apex oriented in a slightly medial direction. However, most Asians have horizontally oriented nostrils. Common rhinoplastic procedures for Asians include changing or correcting this shape. Possible factors affecting nostril shape include characteristics of the alar cartilage, nasal tip supporting structures, and pull of nasal muscles on the surrounding the area. Although a distinct anatomy for each structure in Asian noses has been described previously, we focus on the relationship of nasal structures with nostril shape.

The dilator naris anterior, dilator naris posterior, and depressor septi nasi muscles are well developed in nostrils with horizontal shape. However, these muscles are poorly developed in vertically oriented nostrils.[20]

Lateral crus shape of the alar cartilage is mostly concave or concave-convex for horizontally oriented nostrils, whereas it is commonly convex or convex-concave for vertically oriented nostrils. Regarding the shape of the medial crus, there is no difference between horizontally and vertically oriented nostrils. Both types have predominantly straight medial crura. However, these two types of nostrils are significantly different in terms of footplate segment ratios. Specifically, horizontally oriented nostrils have greater footplate segment ratios in the medial crus than vertically oriented nostrils.[20]

Based on the anatomic differences between horizontally and vertically oriented nostrils, a more aesthetically pleasing nostril shape may be achieved by weakening dilator naris anterior, dilator naris posterior, and depressor septi nasi muscles. Another method involves altering the lateral crus shape through cartilage suture techniques. Finally, changing the footplate segment ratio is accomplished by transferring part of the footplate segment to the columellar segment through a footplate approximation to produce an acceptable nostril shape.[1,20,34]

EXTERNAL NASAL NERVE

The external nasal branch of the anterior ethmoidal nerve (or external nasal nerve) emerges between the nasal bone and the upper lateral cartilage. The external nasal nerve is wholly sensory and is often severed during endonasal incisions or dissections around the rhinion. Transection of the external nasal nerve results in numbness of the nasal tip. However, this is not usually detected during surgical procedure. The numbness or hypoesthesia likely causes a great deal of inconvenience to patients. It may produce permanent loss of sensation or paresthesias over the nasal tip portion.[35,36] In addition, some patients have complaints of neuralgic pain or severe hyperesthesias that can start several months after the surgery because of stump neuroma formation.[35,37,38] This complication has occasionally been the subject of litigation, and it is likely underdiagnosed.[39] Thus, surgeons who perform the rhinoplasty should be familiar with the anatomy of this nerve.

The exit point of the external nasal nerve from the distal nasal bone is fairly consistently located 6.5 mm to 8.5 mm (mean, 7.3 mm) lateral to the nasal midline regardless of the size of the nasal bone (**Fig. 8**). The average diameter of the nerve at the point of exit is 0.4 mm. After emerging from a small groove in the distal nasal bone, the external nasal nerve passes into the deep fatty layer directly beneath the superficial musculoaponeurotic layer.[40]

The following suggestions minimize injury to this nerve in Asian rhinoplasty. First, it is best to

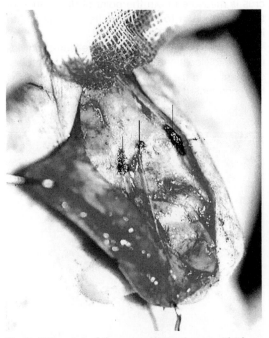

Fig. 8. Exit point of the external nasal nerve. Thick arrow indicates the point of exit of the nerve. Thin arrows indicate nasal midline and nasomaxillary suture.

avoid deep intercartilaginous or intracartilaginous incisions. Instead, dissections should be maintained directly on the surface of the cartilage (deep to the deep fatty layer). Second, soft tissue dissection at the junction of the nasal bone and upper lateral cartilage area should not extend too far laterally. It should be limited within 6.5 mm from the midline of each side. Lastly, when the nasal dorsum is augmented by an onlay graft, implants or graft materials less than 13 mm in width at rhinion level should be used exclusively.[40]

BLOOD SUPPLY OF THE NASAL TIP

The nasal superficial arterial system is well known based on various anatomic investigations. In Asians, vascular research of the nose has focused on blood supply of the nasal tip because the use of open rhinoplasty approach or tip debulking procedure is increased. This can raise the possibility of skin necrosis at the nasal tip. Cases of nasal tip deformity caused by scar contracture have also been observed.

According to studies on white cadavers, the main blood supply of the nasal tip is fulfilled by the lateral nasal artery. Therefore, there is little risk of tip necrosis, even when the columella artery is severed.[41–43] Jung and colleagues[44] have reported that main vessels are distributed at the nasal tip and columella in Asians. The lateral nasal artery is the main blood supply to the nasal tip in 78% of cases, whereas the dorsal nasal artery is the main blood supply to the nasal tip in 22% of cases. The lateral or dorsal nasal artery supplies the nasal tip via the nasal SMAS layer or the superficial fat layer directly above it. This artery passes the dome region of the alar cartilage that determines the tip-defining point. Therefore, it is easily injured during surgical dissection of this area. The distance between the alar groove and the lateral nasal artery has been reported to be 3 mm in white persons. However, it is measured to be 4 mm in Asians.

REFERENCES

1. Han SK, Woo HS, Kim WK. Extended incision in open-approach rhinoplasty for Asians. Plast Reconstr Surg 2002;109:2087–96.
2. McKinney P, Sweis I. A clinical definition of an ideal nasal radix. Plast Reconstr Surg 2002;109:1416–8 [discussion: 1419–20].
3. Jang YJ, Alfanta EM. Rhinoplasty in the Asian nose. Facial Plast Surg Clin North Am 2014;22:357–77.
4. Ishii CH. Current update in Asian rhinoplasty. Plast Reconstr Surg Glob Open 2014;2:e133.
5. Jang YJ, Moon BJ. State of the art in augmentation rhinoplasty: implant or graft? Curr Opin Otolaryngol Head Neck Surg 2012;20:280–6.
6. Zelken JA, Hong JP, Broyles JM, et al. Preventing elevated radix deformity in Asian rhinoplasty with a chimeric dorsal-glabellar construct. Aesthet Surg J 2016;36:287–96.
7. Yu MS, Jang YJ. Preoperative computer simulation for Asian rhinoplasty patients: analysis of accuracy and patient preference. Aesthet Surg J 2014;34:1162–71.
8. Fitzgerald JP, Nanda RS, Currier GF. An evaluation of the nasolabial angle and the relative inclinations of the nose and upper lip. Am J Orthod Dentofacial Orthop 1992;102:328–34.
9. Legan HL, Burstone CJ. Soft tissue cephalometric analysis for orthognathic surgery. J Oral Surg 1980;38:744–51.
10. Nandini S, Prashanth CS, Somiah SK, et al. An evaluation of nasolabial angle and the relative inclinations of the nose and upper lip. J Contemp Dent Pract 2011;12:152–7.
11. Armijo BS, Brown M, Guyuron B. Defining the ideal nasolabial angle. Plast Reconstr Surg 2012;129:759–64.
12. Biller JA, Kim DW. A contemporary assessment of facial aesthetic preferences. Arch Facial Plast Surg 2009;11:91–7.
13. Sinno HH, Markarian MK, Ibrahim AM, et al. The ideal nasolabial angle in rhinoplasty: a preference analysis of the general population. Plast Reconstr Surg 2014;134:201–10.
14. Monasterio FO, Orsini R. Surgery of the non-Indo-European face. Clin Plast Surg 1996;23:341–56.
15. Kim NG, Park SW, Park HO, et al. Are differences in external noses between whites and Koreans caused by differences in the nasal septum? J Craniofac Surg 2015;26:922–6.
16. Cho GS, Kim JH, Yeo NK, et al. Nasal skin thickness measured using computed tomography and its effect on tip surgery outcomes. Otolaryngol Head Neck Surg 2011;144:522–7.
17. Han SK. Asian rhinoplasty. Seoul (South Korea): Koonja Publishing Inc; 2006.
18. Tansatit T, Moon HJ, Rungsawang C, et al. Safe planes for injection rhinoplasty: a histological analysis of midline longitudinal sections of the Asian nose. Aesthetic Plast Surg 2016;40:236–44.
19. Chun KW, Kang HJ, Han SK, et al. Anatomy of the alar lobule in the Asian nose. J Plast Reconstr Aesthet Surg 2008;61:400–7.
20. Ducut EG, Han SK, Kim SB, et al. Factors affecting nostril shape in Asian noses. Plast Reconstr Surg 2006;118:1613–21 [discussion: 1622–3].
21. Jung JA, Jung SY, Han SK, et al. Nostrilplasty by manipulating the dilator naris muscles: a pilot study. Plast Reconstr Surg 2016;138:1010–3.

22. Han SK, Lee DG, Kim JB, et al. An anatomic study of nasal tip supporting structures. Ann Plast Surg 2004;52:134–9.

23. Han SK, Ko HW, Lee DY, et al. The effect of releasing tip-supporting structures in short-nose correction. Ann Plast Surg 2005;54:375–8.

24. Han SK, Jeong SH, Lee BI, et al. Updated anatomy of the dermocartilaginous ligament of the nose. Ann Plast Surg 2007;59:393–7.

25. Lee CH, Han SK, Kim SB, et al. Augmentation rhinoplasty minimizing nasion level changes: a simple method. Plast Reconstr Surg 2008;121:334e–5e.

26. Pitanguy I, Salgado F, Radwanski HN, et al. The surgical importance of the dermocartilaginous ligament of the nose. Plast Reconstr Surg 1995;95:790–4.

27. Zelnik J, Gingrass RP. Anatomy of the alar cartilage. Plast Reconstr Surg 1979;64:650–3.

28. Ofodile FA, James EA. Anatomy of alar cartilages in blacks. Plast Reconstr Surg 1997;100:699–703.

29. Dhong ES, Han SK, Lee CH, et al. Anthropometric study of alar cartilage in Asians. Ann Plast Surg 2002;48:386–91.

30. Sheen JH, Sheen AP. Applied anatomy and physiology. Aesthetic rhinoplasty. 2nd edition. St Louis (MO): Mosby; 1987. p. 25–45.

31. Guyuron B. Precision rhinoplasty. Part I: the role of life-size photographs and soft-tissue cephalometric analysis. Plast Reconstr Surg 1988;81:489–99.

32. Sajjadian A, Rubinstein R, Naghshineh N. Current status of grafts and implants in rhinoplasty: part I. Autologous grafts. Plast Reconstr Surg 2010;125:40e–9e.

33. Kim JS, Khan NA, Song HM, et al. Intraoperative measurements of harvestable septal cartilage in rhinoplasty. Ann Plast Surg 2010;65:519–23.

34. Han SK, Ko HW, Kim WK. Advantages of adding a footplate incision in Asian rhinoplasty. Ann Plast Surg 2004;53:65–9.

35. Thompson AC. Nasal tip numbness following rhinoplasty. Clin Otolaryngol Allied Sci 1987;12:143–4.

36. Bafaqeeh SA, al-Qattan MM. Alterations in nasal sensibility following open rhinoplasty. Br J Plast Surg 1998;51:508–10.

37. Golding-Wood DG, Brookes GB. Post-traumatic external nasal neuralgia–an often missed cause of facial pain? Postgrad Med J 1991;67:55–6.

38. Drysdale AJ, Moore-Gillon V. External nasal nerve division: a treatment for post-traumatic neuralgia. J Laryngol Otol 1992;106:915–6.

39. McKinney P, Cook JQ. A critical evaluation of 200 rhinoplasties. Ann Plast Surg 1981;7:357–61.

40. Han SK, Shin YW, Kim WK. Anatomy of the external nasal nerve. Plast Reconstr Surg 2004;114:1055–9.

41. Rohrich RJ, Gunter JP, Friedman RM. Nasal tip blood supply: an anatomic study validating the safety of the transcolumellar incision in rhinoplasty. Plast Reconstr Surg 1995;95:795–9 [discussion: 800–1].

42. Toriumi DM, Mueller RA, Grosch T, et al. Vascular anatomy of the nose and the external rhinoplasty approach. Arch Otolaryngol Head Neck Surg 1996;122:24–34.

43. Hassard AD, Holness RO. The "crossbow" incision and nasal flap–its blood supply and clinical application. Head Neck Surg 1984;7:135–8.

44. Jung DH, Kim HJ, Koh KS, et al. Arterial supply of the nasal tip in Asians. Laryngoscope 2000;110:308–11.

Hybrid Approach for Asian Rhinoplasty
Open Approach Without Transcolumellar Incision

Jae-Goo Kang, MD, PhD[a],*, Kyung Won Kwon, MD[a],
Jinsoon Chang, MD, PhD[b]

KEYWORDS

- Open approach without transcolumellar incision • Modified septal extension graft
- Approach for Asian rhinoplasty • Nonopen approach

KEY POINTS

- An essential merit of endonasal rhinoplasty is the ability of the surgeon to fine-tune the nasal shape from intact skin, which is not always possible with the open approach.
- The hybrid approach (open approach without transcolumellar incision) delivers unlimited exposure and technical access, enabling all the procedures possible in the open approach while offering the surface feedback of endonasal surgery.
- The hybrid approach follows the same logic, sequence, and techniques of the open structural rhinoplasty, putting great emphasis on gaining maximal access to the skeleton.
- The hybrid approach also enables both a left-brain mode of operation (analysis and technical precision; from open access to the anatomy) and right-brain mode of surgery (appreciation of shape, balance, or proportion from intact skin).
- Technically, only the marginal incisions are required for the open approach.

INTRODUCTION
Is the Endonasal Approach Working for Asian Noses?

Contemporary endonasal rhinoplasty has broadened its indications and now embraces maneuvers that are typically reserved for an open approach.[1–3] The infracartilaginous approach allows technical access for most tip-modifying maneuvers.[4] More complex and profound changes of the lower lateral cartilage (LLC), such as medial advancement of the dome and lateral crural strut, are performed from complete release of the lateral crus via endonasal approach.[5] The transvestibular approach of Fuleihan[6] is a recent addition of endonasal expansion, giving improved access and manipulation of the LLC through the transvestibular dissection.

Nonetheless, all of these approaches share essential ingredients of endonasal rhinoplasty: respect or preserve the innate tip support mechanism of the medial crura, and disrupt the medial crura or skin attachment as minimally as possible.[7] The advantages stemming from this are multiple: less surgery, less morbidity, and less graft requirement, while offering an equivalent (if not superior) and quicker outcome. Preservation of the natural softness of the tip is appreciable on

Disclosure Statement: The authors have nothing to disclose.
[a] Department of Otolaryngology–Head and Neck Surgery, National Medical Center, Ulchiro 245, Choong-Gu, Seoul 04564, Korea; [b] Department of Otolaryngology–Head and Neck Surgery, Inje University Seoul Paik Hospital, Seoul, Korea
* Corresponding author.
E-mail address: kwilly@daum.net

Facial Plast Surg Clin N Am 26 (2018) 269–283
https://doi.org/10.1016/j.fsc.2018.03.002

the postoperative visit, attesting to the real merit and elegance of the endonasal surgery.

However, these endonasal benefits are not available for every nose. What if there are substantial problems in the sacred region, the columellar anatomy? These include

1. Severe deficiencies of medial crural support
2. Major asymmetries in the medial crura, such as in cleft deformities.

Even advocates of endonasal surgery prefer an open approach for direct repair of deficient medial crura and the use of grafts to attain a well-supported and aesthetic nasal tip.[8-10] It is inevitable the nose be opened if the surgeon wants a precise correction of the deficient anatomy. However, in the open approach, the surgeon loses not only the inherent tip support but also the most precious advantage of endonasal rhinoplasty: the opportunity to see the undisturbed surface and, hence, fine-tune or control the nasal shape. Endonasal rhinoplasty is an operation designed so that intraoperative skin surface changes can be observed, providing appropriate feedback for subsequent decisions.[7] However, the weak or deficient medial crura of Asian noses (**Fig. 1**A) do not permit using this endonasal merit. Surgeons must expose or manipulate the medial crura, thus losing the surface control of endonasal surgery. It seems unavoidable; however, there is a way to retain this endonasal merit (availability of the surface feedback) while performing a complete dissection of open rhinoplasty.

An Open Approach Without Opening the Nose

The approach reported by Guerrerosantos and echoed by other surgeons[11-13] is essentially an open approach without transcolumellar incision, as its name implies. It is not a wider dissection version of endonasal surgery because there is little respect for basic endonasal tenets (limited dissection, pocket-grafting, and minimizing inadvertent loss of supporting system). Instead, it follows the same logic, sequence, and techniques of open structural rhinoplasty (OSR), placing great emphasis on gaining maximal access to the skeleton.[14-16] Its emergence was prompted by the same demand of open rhinoplasty for increased surgical versatility and technical accuracy.

As shown in the figures in this article, excellent visualization of this approach allows virtually all the procedures possible in the open approach: manipulation on the entire septal strut (spreader graft and correction of the caudal septum) and various surgical techniques on the nasal tip (cephalic resection, lateral crural flap, sutures, or graft placement). It really is an open approach, having the same precision and surgical control (**Fig. 1**B). The difference from the open approach is that it avoids transcolumellar incision and retains skin continuity throughout the entire operation. This difference is not merely sparing 1 incision but provides the surgeon a significant benefit: the unique opportunity to control surface change in real time

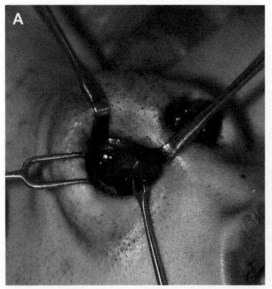
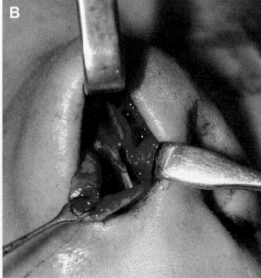

Fig. 1. (*A*) Medial crura of Asian noses demand an open exposure for direct repair and support of the weak or deficient anatomy. (*B*) The hybrid approach delivers unlimited exposure and technical access, comparable to an open approach.

on every step of rhinoplasty. This approach is an unusual gift to rhinoplasty surgeons, enabling both a left-brain mode of operation (analysis and technical precision; from open access to the anatomy) and a right-brain mode of surgery (appreciation of shape, balance, or proportion in overall context of the nose, **Fig. 2**).

Technically, only the marginal incisions are required for this approach.[17] The key to gaining wide-exposure (see **Fig. 1**) is

1. Extension of the incisions down to the foot plate of the medial crura
2. Complete separation of the LLC from its retaining forces and complete dissection of the membranous septum to get its comfortable delivery and manipulation.

See later discussion of the detailed technical aspects.

PERTINENT SURGICAL ANATOMY: OPERATIVE PHILOSOPHY

Contrary to Western rhinoplasty in which the direction of surgery is mainly reductive (to get a smaller version of a refined nose), the direction is quite opposite in Asian patients in whom it is augmentative to get more projection. The open approach is the rule to get maximum exposure and technical access for various grafting requirements.[18,19]

Anatomic Handicap of Asian Noses Favors the Septal Extension Graft, Hence the Open Approach

An inverse relationship between the thickness of the skin and of the thickness of the LLC is generally true, and source of poor tip definition and suboptimal outcome of tip surgery on Asian patients. Reduction of the LLC in an attempt to refine the tip leads to even more amorphous shape and projection loss.[20,21] The thick skin–soft tissue envelope of Asian nose prevents contraction. Wishful thinking of tip refinement through removal of the LLC ends up with a scar forming between the recalcitrant skin envelope and surgically diminished LLC. To overcome this hurdle, Asian nasal tips conversely need more structures to project through the thicker skin, thereby gaining a visible refinement. This means not only more cartilage grafts but also more stable methods of support to the tip structures than that normally used (columellar strut) used in tip surgery for white patients.[17]

The columellar strut results in an upturned, overrotated tip when one tries to produce a greater projection gain, using the strut.[19] Undoubtedly, special measures are required to prevent this

rotation of the nasal tip. Augmentation in most Asian cases requires some lengthening, not just projection of the nose (see **Fig. 2**). Technically, caudal advancement as well as projection of the nasal tip complex, is an important surgical task. The septal extension graft (SEG) has become a preferred tool to achieve this goal. The SEG is a truly versatile technique that controls tip projection or rotation, the alar–columella relationship, and the shape of the nasolabial angle.

The following characteristics are well-known handicaps of the Asian nasal tip, inaccessible and neglected in the past[22]:

- Short or retracted columella with premaxilla hypoplasia
- Transverse nostril, often with alar notching
- Skin–soft tissue envelope, unyielding to tip sculpting
- Underprojected tip, prone to rotation.

This can be managed with SEG, providing a solid and firm foundation and the favorable tip position required for Asian noses. When the SEG is sutured into position, the alar cartilages are moved up on the extension graft, constituting another reason to use an open approach in Asian noses.

Adequate Release of the Lower Lateral Cartilage Is Critical, Which Sets up the Open Structural Rhinoplasty

Substantial projection and caudal movement of the LLC is usually required for the desired tip position. This causes undue tension, which in turn compromises the long-term maintenance of nasal tip position.[23,24] Therefore, adequate mobilization and release of the LLC from its retaining forces (at the scroll and the hinge region) is most critical to successful LLC repositioning (**Figs. 3** and **4**)[25]:

- Release at the scroll area assists derotation (caudal movement of LLC)
- Nasal hinge release allows better tip projection (anterior movement of LLC).

The extent of dissection no longer belongs in endonasal surgery. Now, it is in OSR, which focuses on

1. Complete exposure and release of the related anatomy (retracted or hypoplastic LLC)
2. Rebuilding with structural reinforcement (SEG as a foundation for nasal tip repositioning).

As such, exclusive use of SEG by means of extended marginal incision becomes the senior author's modus operandi for tip surgery on Asian patients.[17]

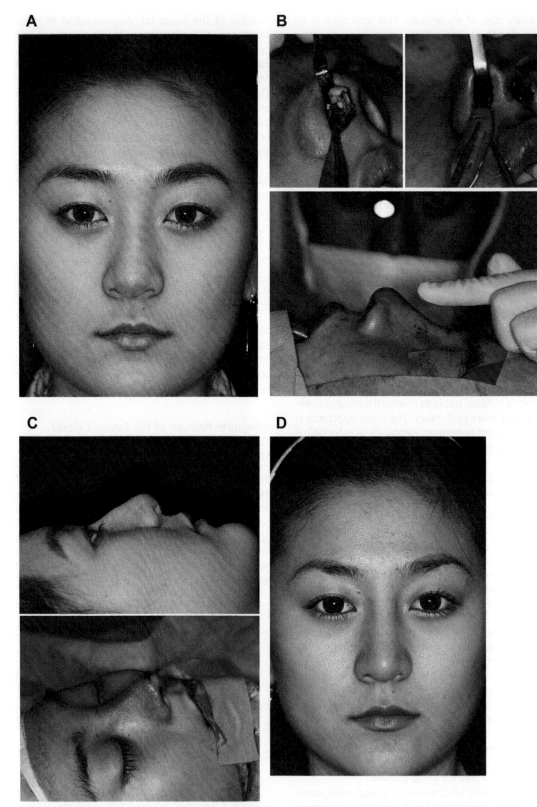

Fig. 2. Available surface feedback from skin continuity of the hybrid approach allows fine-tuning of minor millimeters of changes on each step of rhinoplasty. (*A*) This is critical when there is great concern over skin sleeve

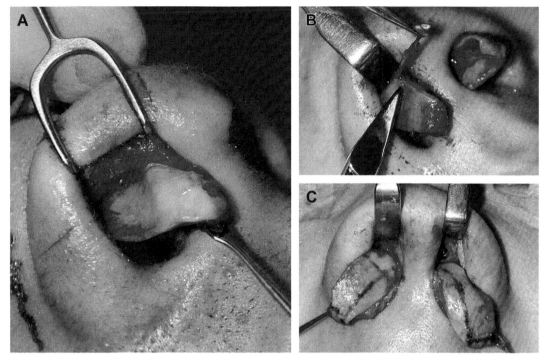

Fig. 3. (*A*) Adequate release of the LLC from its retaining forces (at the scroll and the hinge region) is most critical step before its tension-free apposition to the SEG. (*B*) Cephalic resection of the LLC should be kept to a minimum and posterior to the dome; its primary purpose is to release the LLC from attachment with the upper lateral cartilage, facilitating caudal movement of the LLC. (*C*) LLC release at the nasal hinge allows its anterior movement.

Avoidance of Columellar Scar Has Particular Benefits in Asian Patients

Although most favored in rhinoplasty on Asian patients, an open approach has shortcomings in thick-skinned patients. The transcolumellar incision can be troublesome and causes an objectionable scar in some patients.[26] There is also an added risk of vascular compromise from defatting procedures, commonly performed on Asian patients.[27,28] Without a doubt, its avoidance is a definite merit in this thick, sebaceous, and dark-skinned population. Though the same can be said for thin-skinned patient, available surface feedback and opportunity for real-time control and adjustment is more precious in tip surgery on Asian patients. This ability, stemming from an intact skin envelope, reduces the vagaries of thicker skin and its intraoperative drapage.[17]

This has been the rationale for the current approach, with special interest for the nasal anatomy of Asian patients; however, the obvious advantages can be shared by all candidates for rhinoplasty of any ethnicity. The senior author recommends this approach be used

1. Whenever OSR offers clear diagnostic and therapeutic advantages (for complex deformity or for technical access)
2. With observation of intraoperative surface change, which is critical owing to the great concern regarding skin sleeve movement, balance change, and the surface effects of each procedure.

OPERATIVE STEPS

The sequence of surgical steps is important and should be designed optimally for improved

movement and balance change as shown in this woman. Refining her large nasal base requires some amount of tip projection, a daunting task in cases where the nasal dorsum is already high enough. (*B*) The hybrid approach enables necessary surface feedback to find an optimal implant width-to-height, as well as tip projection. (*C*) Immediate outcome on the operating table in comparison with preoperative profile. (*D*) On postoperative frontal view. Her nose looks smaller and narrower even though her nasal dimension increased from tip projection or dorsal augmentation. The hybrid approach allowed right-brain mode surgery to achieve successful balancing between the upper and lower nose in this challenging case.

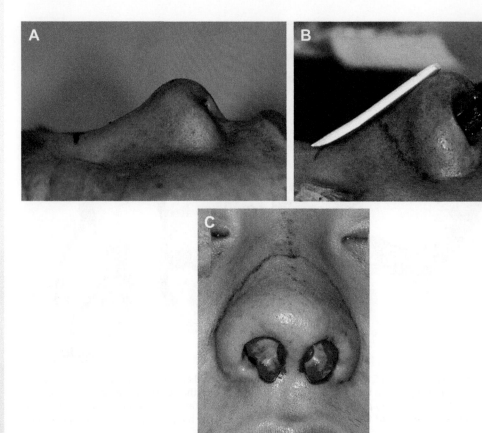

Fig. 4. (*A*) A young gentleman with short and up-turned nasal profile. (*B*) Substantial advancement of LLC is shown after its release, profile view. (*C*) Anterior view of the same patient.

control, less risk of over operation, and less risk of a maneuver having adverse effects on another previously modified area. The optimal sequence varies with the approach itself but it also depends on the surgical contents; for example, whether it is primarily reductive or augmentative.[7,20]

Distinctive merits of the current approach allow diverse indications of its use: narrowing of the bulbous tip (**Fig. 5**), lengthening of the overrotated tip (**Fig. 6**), improvement of alar–columella disharmony, and correction of the deviated nose (**Fig. 7**). It is certainly beneficial for challenging cases of endonasal of rhinoplasty on White patients. However, in this context and patient population, it seems suitable to limit the operative scope to augmentation rhinoplasty on Asian patients to best illustrate the surgical steps with logical and proper sequence.

Access Incisions

The initial marginal incision begins at the soft tissue facet and proceeds laterally as far as the posterior tip of the lateral crus. Then, the senior author reverses the direction of the No. 15 blade to incise medially from the apex past the columella and extend farther down to the footplate of the medial crura (**Fig. 8**A). An identical incision is made on the opposite side.

This extended marginal incision should be long enough because this is the only access incision for delivery of the alar cartilage, as well as exposure of the entire septum or upper lateral complex and the bony pyramids. When alar batten grafts are planned, the lateral extent of the marginal incision is limited so that a virginal pocket for a batten graft is preserved.

Delivery of the Alar Cartilage and Primary Release of the Lower Lateral Cartilage (at the Scroll)

Using small curved scissors, the nasal tip skin is separated from the LLC. This dissection starts from the posterior margin of the LLC and extends past and medially to the dome. The second dissection pocket is developed at the columellar limb of the incision. Sharp dissection is preferred to maintain the integrity of thin columellar skin but remain caudal to the medial crura. Proactive

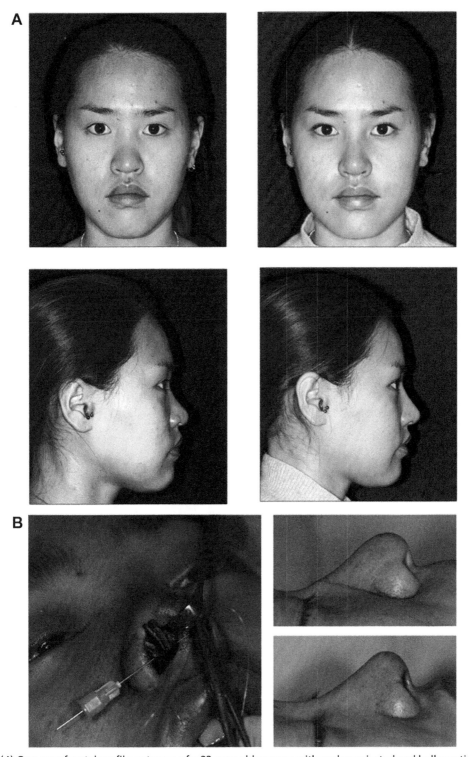

Fig. 5. (*A*) One-year frontal profile outcome of a 23-year-old woman with underprojected and bulbous tip, using SEG as supporting grafts via the hybrid approach. (*B*) The wide-field dissection of the hybrid approach facilitates complete exposure and sutures for the extension graft, yet enables delicate control of the nasal shape with the intact skin envelop.

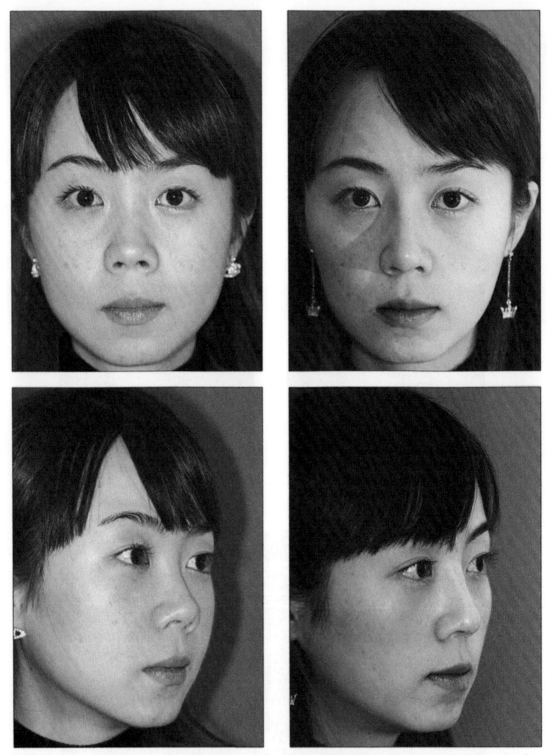

Fig. 6. Outcome of the hybrid approach in conjunction with a modified SEG in a 20-year-old woman with a fore-shortened overrotated tip.

identification of its caudal margin prevents its damage. Then, the 2 pockets are connected, which is facilitated by caudal traction of the dome with a single skin hook (**Fig. 8**B).

Next, each LLC can be pulled out of the nostril and the exposure is no less than that of the delivery approach. Cephalic resection is performed and should be kept minimal and posterior to the

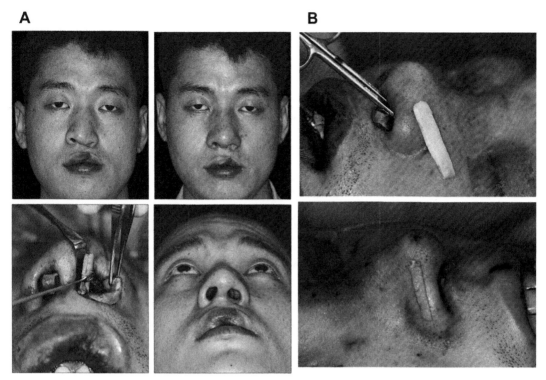

Fig. 7. (*A*) Outcome of the hybrid approach in a patient with a secondary cleft-lip nose deformity, showing excellent visualization for complex maneuvers such as costal cartilage extension graft and lateral crural strut. (*B*) Dimension and position of a long lateral crural strut used in this patient. Alar rim grafting via the hybrid approach in another case. Hypoplastic or cephalically malpositioned LLC of Asian noses requires support in the alar wall as much as to the central nasal tip.

dome because its primary purpose is to release the LLC from attachment with the upper lateral cartilage, never to reduce the volume (see **Fig. 3**). The vestibular lining is always preserved. Some midline fibrous connections with skin envelope often remain near the surface of the dome. Cutting these connections completes its separation from the tip skin and prepares for the next step.

Dissection of the Membranous Septum and Exposure of the Caudal Margin of the Septum

To gain access to the caudal septum, further dissection is required. Deliver the fully mobilized LLC into 1 nostril. Separation of the LLCs from each other begins at the interdomal ligament, and proceeds inferiorly and posteriorly in a top-down manner (**Fig. 8**C). Under direct vision, sharp dissection is performed in the precise midline of the membranous septum, which can be aided by lateral traction of the LLCs from each other (opening up the potential dissecting plane). In some severely crooked noses, the caudal margin of the septum can be quite off the midline. It is easy to lose the precise dissection plane and perforate

the membranous septum. Vigilant palpation and confirming the position of the caudal margin is crucial to avoid such mishap. As such, complete exposure of the entire caudal septum plus anterior nasal spine is achieved (**Fig. 8**D). At this stage, the entire LLC can be delivered to each nostril, permitting simultaneous visualization of both alar cartilages without distortion, which is not allowed in an endonasal approach (**Fig. 8**E). In purely cosmetic cases with a straight septum, in which the role of septoplasty is confined to graft harvest, the access to the septum is gained through a separate hemitransfixion incision. To preserve the strength and integrity of the caudal septum, dissection of the entire membranous septum is avoided and the connection between the posterior septal angle and the membranous septum remains virgin.

Skeletonization of the Dorsum, Septal Correction, and Harvest or Osteotomy

For skeletonization of the dorsum, septal correction, and harvest or osteotomy procedures, there is no unique point of the current approach requiring special description. Surgical exposures,

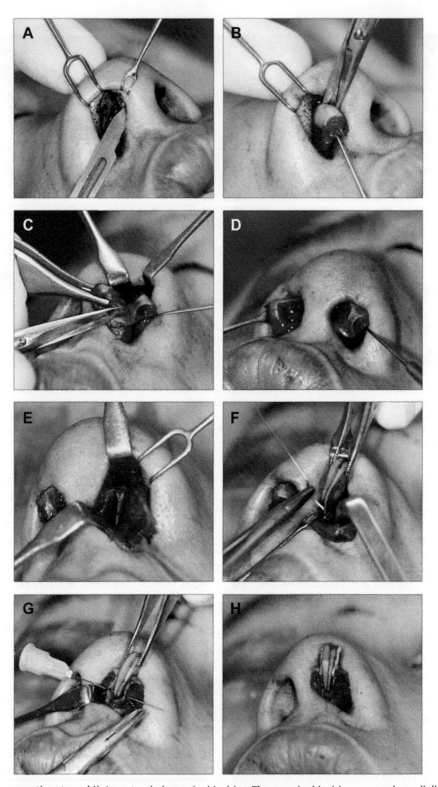

Fig. 8. Intraoperative steps. (*A*) An extended marginal incision The marginal incision proceeds medially past the columella and extends down to the footplate of the medial crura. (*B*) Delivery of the alar cartilage. Dissection beginning at the lateral portion of the LLC is connected to the medial dissection pocket at the columellar limb of the incision. This is facilitated by caudal traction of the dome with a single skin hook. (*C*) Dissection of the

and the content and maneuverability of technical procedures, are almost identical to the open approach.[29] The order of procedures is given in the following sections.

Skeletonization and removal of the dorsal hump

Septal correction and harvest Unlike the open approach, technical access can be somewhat limited with placement of the suture-secured spreader grafts, especially in patients who have a tight skin envelope. Enthusiastic septal harvesting (remaining width of caudal strut <10 mm) can handicap septal integrity, causing postoperative problems. One should always leave at least a 12-mm width strut caudally and dorsally.

Osteotomies The need for bilateral osteotomies in rhinoplasty on an Asian patient is generally uncommon. Planned dorsal augmentation favors wider dorsal platform, so indiscreet osteotomies are only counterproductive, creating unnatural stepladders in the side wall.

Because the dorsal profile and axial alignment is settled, attention is shifted to the nasal tip.

Placement of Septal Extension Graft

The harvested septum is cut into the SEG. Life-size images are used in preoperative planning.[17] A precise SEG is cut using a previously crafted paper template. Markings for anchoring points of the alar cartilage and overlapping the caudal septum are precisely transferred. Appropriate traction with 2 small blunt retractors can fully expose the caudal septum and provide enough working space for placing the SEG (**Fig. 8F**). The SEG is inserted precisely at the planned position on the septum, usually with 3 5-0 polydioxanone (PDS) sutures. Precise positioning of the SEG is the most critical step of the nasal tip surgery because its caudal margin forms the actual nasal tip shape (**Box 1**).

From the intact skin envelope, precise control of the tip-position can be executed in the most accurate and efficient manner, which is not available in the open approach. Two types of SEG are preferably used and described in the senior author's (Kang and Ryu[17]) previous paper.

Repositioning of the Lower Lateral Cartilage

To reposition of the LLC, the affixed extension graft and both alar cartilages are delivered to 1 side and the alar cartilages are sutured exactly at the anchoring points marked on the extension graft, using 5-0 PDS sutures, first at the columellar break point and second at the cephalic dome (see **Fig. 8G**).[17] Placement of the dome suture at the cephalic dome is important for proper orientation of the lateral crus. This is done by lowering its cephalic margin while elevating its caudal margin, thereby reducing possible supratip rounding and supporting the alar margin.[29]

Dismantling all retaining components of the LLC before suturing it to the SEG is an essential step, as previously discussed. Release in the scroll area was performed in the previous step of alar cartilage delivery. For its anterior advancement (projection), deeper dissection is required to release the LLC (at the scroll and nasal hinge) for comfortable and tension-free apposition to the SEG. From the senior authors' clinical observation, the pyriform ligament is composed of multiple layers of tissue. During its dissection, the possibility of mucosal tear should always be considered and excessive release is not recommended.

Dorsal Augmentation

For ordinary cases, alloplastic (Silastics [AART Inc, Reno, Nevada] or Goretex [W. L. Gore & Associates Inc, Flagstaff, Arizona]) is preferred. During refinement of the nasal tip, the dorsal graft is repeatedly removed and inserted to adjust its

---

membranous septum to expose the caudal margin of the septum. After delivering both alar cartilages into 1 nostril, separation of the LLCs from each other begins at the interdomal ligament and proceeds inferiorly and posteriorly in a top-down manner. Under direct vision, sharp dissection is performed in the precise midline of the membranous septum. (*D*) Visualization of undistorted nasal tip anatomy. The entire LLC can be delivered to each nostril, permitting simultaneous visualization of both alar cartilages without distortion. This is not available in the endonasal approach, in which the membranous septum is not dissected. (*E*) Exposure of the caudal septum. Careful midline dissection and vigilant palpation of the caudal septum is essential to avoid perforating the membranous septum. The resulting exposure includes complete visualization of the entire septal strut plus anterior nasal spine. (*F*) Placement of SEG. The dissected caudal septum is fully exposed with 2 blunt retractors. The extension graft overlaps and is sutured to the caudal septum at the desired position. (*G*) Repositioning of the alar cartilage. After adequate mobilization of the LLC, both alar cartilages are delivered to the left nostril and sutured to the extension graft, first at the columellar break point and second at the cephalic dome. (*H*) Procuring adequate width and refinement of the nasal tip. Additional cartilage battens are sutured on either side of the projected portion of the extension graft to secure an adequate tip width. The leading edge of the tip complex of 7 to 9 mm thickness is further camouflaged by thin layers of perichondrium.

width and relationship with the tip projection. Thorough disinfection measures should be exercised: intranasal prep with povidone iodine, periodic cleansing of the wound with saline irrigation, covering the patient's mouth prior to suture-entering surgical field, changing gloves, and minimizing handling of alloplastic.

Refinement of the Nasal Tip

To secure adequate width of the natural-appearing nasal tip, cartilage battens are attached to the SEG (**Fig. 8**H).[25] The leading edge of the tip complex is 7 to 9 mm thick and composed of quadruples of septal or ear cartilage. Thin layers of perichondrium further camouflage the tip complex. The sewn cartilage complex is put back into the skin cover and examined, then meticulously carved to achieve the desired appearance. To make this decision, the following questions should be considered:

1. Is the tip lobule symmetrical or irregular? Does the tip profile still look good?
2. Does the width of the nasal tip blend with the dorsal aesthetic line?
3. Is there a deep supra-alar crease or tendency of notching nostril that calls for grafting (for external valve support)?
4. Are there any final touches necessary in the tip appearance?

The answers for these questions are

1. The nasal tip complex is carefully examined under the skin cover for its symmetry and irregularities. A slight supratip-depression and bottom-heavy nasal tip lobule (the mass of the lobule falls caudal to the peak projection, pronasale) is preferred.[30] If the vertical dimension of the supratip lobule appears high in the profile view, forming a rounded look at the supratip, drag back the tip complex into the nostril and reduce its cephalic mass.
2. For confluent brow-dome lines, the width of the nasal tip complex (quadruples of cartilage) is adjusted or width of the dorsal graft is adjusted. If there is some depression in the supratip region, crushed cartilage is placed over the area as camouflage filler.
3. During the refinement stage of the nasal tip, it is quite common to encounter external valve issues such as a deepened supra-alar crease (from poor alar wall support) and nostril retraction.[31] Preexisting conditions such as nostril notching or prominent alar crease are aggravated from common tip procedures (cephalic trim, interdomal sutures, and alar base

---

Box 1
Expanded usage of the septal extension graft: combing a tip graft with a supporting graft

The SEG is a supporting graft and a hidden graft (which does not show externally). Its use can be expanded to form a nasal tip lobule by adding length and converting it from a hidden graft to a projecting graft. If one looks closely at the shape of the SEG in **Fig. 8**H, there is some extra length, protruding over to the existing dome. The reasons for this extra length are numerous.

PRECISE CONTROL OF THE NASAL TIP PROFILE

Modified use of the protruding component of the SEG enables precise realization of a preplanned tip profile. This modification renders the situation exactly the same as preparing an exact dorsal graft that matches preplanned target profile from life-size images. In the senior author's precision rhinoplasty, a template accurately reflecting the target tip profile is prepared in the preoperative stage, using life-size images, which the senior author uses to craft an exact SEG during the operation (see **Fig. 8**).

MORE EFFICIENT NASAL TIP SURGERY, BOTH IN GRAFT-NEED AND IN STRATEGY

In almost all Asian rhinoplasties, shield-type tip grafts are used over the alar complex. Native alar cartilages are often too weak to express a sculpted tip and are concealed under thicker skin, hence they serve merely as a platform for the tip grafts. A second tip graft is a frequent request as a buttress graft to support the shield graft. Use of a third graft is not unusual. More grafts introduce more variables and complicates nasal tip-shaping. This is unnecessary in the senior author's nasal tip strategy. A single graft (modified SEG) forms the nasal tip, providing a simple yet precise shaping and more economic use of the valuable cartilage, so more is available for other uses.

OPTIMAL CONTROL OF THE NOSTRIL-TO-LOBULE RATIO

If surgeons try to achieve nasal tip projection only with the SEG (without additional tip grafts), it frequently leads to a large nostril to small tip disproportion. Their innate deficiency of intrinsic tip component (dimension and strength of the middle crus) does not match the increased columellar length gained from SEG. A balanced outcome requires additional grafts to expand the tip lobule. With a modified SEG, the nostril-to-lobule ratio is readily controlled by regulating the pinning point of medial crura or middle crura-junction on the SEG (see **Fig. 5**B).

resections). Nearing the end of operation, this becomes more intensified with the SEG. The alar rim appears more retracted and more collapsed whereas the central nasal tip looks overemphasized with the SEG, resulting in an unnatural snarl-like nose or sharp interruption between the nasal tip and the alar lobule. This is not a surprising outcome for the LLC anatomy of Asian patients who are handicapped by the double whammy of being hypoplastic and being malpositioned cephalically. Most noses show cephalic malposition of the LLC, which is the rule rather than the exception in this population. Some surgeons have an optimistic view and trust that their thicker skin provides enough alar support, hence further support to the alar wall is not necessary. Biological rules tell it differently: unsupported soft tissue contracts and contracted tissue thickens, thicker skin requires stronger support, not less.[7] The senior author strongly believes this after seeing more and more problems in the sidewall aesthetics of the nasal tip and an increasing need for correction in this area.

Methods to support the sidewall of the nasal ala, includes:

Alar rim graft
  For minor cases of retraction on alar rim support
Lateral crural onlay
  To provide smooth transition from the nasal tip to the alar wall
  Used when projection of the graft-end over the existing dome exceeds 3 mm[29]
Alar batten
  To support the intervalve area beneath the supra-alar crease
  The pocket needs to be precisely the same size as the graft for its retentive quality
Lateral crural underlay (alar strut)
  Not commonly performed and reserved for a significant nostril retraction, not focal retraction
  Powerful enough to create deformities, such as asymmetry in the alar wall or nostril shape
  Composite graft is favored in the presence of vestibular lining defects.
4. On closing incisions with 6-0 nylon sutures, inspect the nasal tip for any nooks and crannies. Small deficiencies can be filled with gently crushed cartilages via the (still) open area in the medial marginal incision.[32] They can be placed in the infratip lobule area or along

the caudal margin of alar complex in the facet region. The cartilage has a soft, spreading, and retentive quality and fills the small gap in and around the tip, ensuring every corner of the recreated surface is well supported.

Again, the availability of direct vision outside is most critical component of this approach. Intraoperative feedback from intact skin allows a delicate touch in evaluating and fine-tuning the final outcome. This offers everything required for precision rhinoplasty by a surgeon with an artistic eye.

PEARLS AND PITFALLS
Pearls

1. On starting dissection at the columellar portion of marginal incision, use very sharp scissors to maintain integrity of thin columellar skin and remain caudal to the medial crura to avoid its damage.
2. During dissection, proactively identify and follow the caudal margin of the LLC. If the caudal margin is lost sight of, find and pick up the posterior part of the lateral crus and dissect retrograde. This is a useful technique in buckled and deformed domal notch of the middle crura.
3. When planning alar batten grafts, the lateral extent of the marginal incision is limited so that a virginal pocket for a batten graft is preserved.
4. In rhinoplasty on Asian patients, the wider field dissection of the current approach necessitates restoring the lost support and more than compensating for it to attain the desired augmentation.
5. Highlights of recent trends and important points in rhinoplasty on Asian patients include
   • The SEG has become a primary tool for Asian nasal tip procedures, producing necessary length as well as projection
   • Challenges of the LLC (hypoplastic or cephalically malpositioned) require the same attention to support the alar wall as to support to central nasal tip (with SEG)
   • Appropriate grafting to support the alar wall produces a natural-looking nasal tip and functional correction of the external valve.
6. Limited graft supply is a practical issue and major restriction in rhinoplasty for Asian patients. Having a precise way to quantitate graft requirements greatly expands the surgeon's control over the outcome by prioritizing available material.

Pitfalls

1. One cannot overcome thick skin by resecting more cartilage from the LLC in an attempt to

get better definition of the nasal tip. On the contrary, thicker skin requires stronger support for its refinement.

2. A tight skin envelope hinders adequate exposure for suturing or grafting, leading to use of undue traction and traumatization of the flap. Rigidly adhering to retaining skin continuity and not opening the nose under such conditions is an altered priority and will set the stage for complications and revisions. Convert to an external columellar incision whenever necessary.

3. An attempt to stretch the limit of the nasal envelope by undue tension with oversized and strong grafts may result in buckling and deflection of the framework, producing both functional and aesthetic problems. Moreover, excessive tension at the incision sites strains survival of the skin flap. In the long term, intended projection and lengthening of the nose may be lost due to graft resorption.

4. In thin-skinned patients, visible prominence, or bossae can be seen postoperatively. The protruding edge of the tip complex should be examined and meticulously carved to avoid any sharp edges and irregularities. Use thin layers of perichondrium to further camouflage the tip complex.

SUMMARY

With the overwhelming popularity of the external approach, surgeons today may not have much exposure to less invasive options. Endonasal rhinoplasty, although not indicated for all patients, is not often used for many qualified Asian candidates. Patients requiring OSR from their significantly handicapped baseline anatomy could be helped with this hybrid approach. In addition, the hybrid approach is flexible in its extent of dissection or exposure. It can be more of a classic-endonasal or limited access approach in some cases or OSR dissection or reconstruction in others. As such, the benefit of nonopen approach deserves equal attention among Asian rhinoplasty surgeons and in residents-in-training courses. The difference is not merely that it spares an incision but it is also an opportunity to fine-tune minor millimeters of changes in every step of rhinoplasty, a real and significant benefit.

REFERENCES

1. Kamer FM, Pieper PG. Nasal tip surgery: a 30-year experience. Facial Plast Surg Clin North Am 2004; 12(1):81–92.
2. Palma P, Khodaei I, Bertossi D, et al. Hybrid rhinoplasty: beyond the dichotomy of rhinoplasty techniques. Acta otorhinolaryngol Ital 2013;33(3): 154–62.
3. Simons RL. Perspectives on the evolution of rhinoplasty. Arch Facial Plast Surg 2009;11(6):409–11.
4. Tasman AJ, Palma P. The infracartilaginous approach revisited. Arch Facial Plast Surg 2008; 10(6):370–5.
5. Gassner HG, Mueller-Vogt U, Strutz J, et al. Nasal tip recontouring in primary rhinoplasty: the endonasal complete release approach. JAMA Facial Plast Surg 2013;15(1):11–6.
6. Fuleihan NS. The transvestibular approach: a new horizon in rhinoplasty. Arch Facial Plast Surg 2006; 8(4):273–82.
7. Constantian MB. Rhinoplasty as an operation. In: Constantian MB, editor. Rhinoplasty: craft and magic. St Louis (MO): Quality Medical; 2009. p. 253–415.
8. Pastorek NJ, Becker DG. Treating the caudal septal deflection. Arch Facial Plast Surg 2000;2(3):217–20.
9. Perkins SW, Tardy ME. External columellar incisional approach to revision of the lower third of the nose. Facial Plast Surg Clin North Am 1993;1:79–98.
10. Perkins SW. The evolution of the combined use of endonasal and external columellar approaches to rhinoplasty. Facial Plast Surg Clin North Am 2004; 12(1):35–50.
11. Guerrerosantos J. Open rhinoplasty without skin-columella incision. Plast Reconstr Surg 1990;85(6): 955–60.
12. Cardenas-Camarena L, Guerrero MT. Improving nasal tip projection and definition using interdomal sutures and open approach without transcolumellar incision. Aesthetic Plast Surg 2002;26(3): 161–6.
13. Bruschi S, Bocchiotti MA, Verga M, et al. Closed rhinoplasty with marginal incision: our experience and results. Aesthetic Plast Surg 2006;30(2):155–8.
14. Toriumi DM. Structure approach in rhinoplasty. Facial Plast Surg Clin North Am 2005;13(1):93–113.
15. Gassner HG. Structural grafts and suture techniques in functional and aesthetic rhinoplasty. GMS Curr Top Otorhinolaryngol Head Neck Surg 2010;9:Doc01.
16. Tebbetts JB. Shaping and positioning the nasal tip without structural disruption: a new, systematic approach. Plast Reconstr Surg 1994;94(1):61–77.
17. Kang JG, Ryu J. Nasal tip surgery using a modified septal extension graft by means of extended marginal incision. Plast Reconstr Surg 2009;123(1):343–52.
18. Jang YJ, Yu MS. Rhinoplasty for the Asian nose. Facial Plast Surg 2010;26(2):93–101.
19. Toriumi DM, Swartout B. Asian rhinoplasty. Facial Plast Surg Clin North Am 2007;15(3):293–307, v.
20. Daniel RK. Secondary rhinoplasty. In: Daniel RK, editor. Rhinoplasty: an atlas of surgical techniques. New York: Springer; 2002. p. 421–525.

21. Pastorek N. Surgical management of the boxy tip. Aesthet Surg J 2007;27(3):306–18 [quiz: 319–21].

22. Lam SM. Asian rhinoplasty. Semin Plast Surg 2009; 23(3):215–22.

23. Jeong JY. Obtaining maximal stability with a septal extension technique in East Asian rhinoplasty. Arch Plast Surg 2014;41(1):19–28.

24. Kim MH, Choi JH, Kim MS, et al. An introduction to the septal extension graft. Arch Plast Surg 2014; 41(1):29–34.

25. Kim JH, Song JW, Park SW, et al. Effective septal extension graft for asian rhinoplasty. Arch Plast Surg 2014;41(1):3–11.

26. Kim HC, Jang YJ. Columellar incision scars in Asian patients undergoing open rhinoplasty. JAMA Facial Plast Surg 2016;18(3):188–93.

27. Bafaqeeh SA, Al-Qattan MM. Simultaneous open rhinoplasty and alar base excision: is there a problem with the blood supply of the nasal tip and columellar skin? Plast Reconstr Surg 2000;105(1):344–7 [discussion: 348–9].

28. Sevin A, Sevin K, Erdogan B, et al. Open rhinoplasty without transcolumellar incision. Ann Plast Surg 2006;57(3):252–4.

29. Toriumi DM. New concepts in nasal tip contouring. Arch Facial Plast Surg 2006;8(3):156–85.

30. Constantian MB. Experience with a three-point method for planning rhinoplasty. Ann Plast Surg 1993;30(1):1–12.

31. Kim EK, Daniel RK. Operative techniques in Asian rhinoplasty. Aesthet Surg J 2012;32(8): 1018–30.

32. Kim JH, Jang YJ. Use of diced conchal cartilage with perichondrial attachment in rhinoplasty. Plast Reconstr Surg 2015;135(6):1545–53.

Augmentation Rhinoplasty Using Silicone Implants

In-Sang Kim, MD

KEYWORDS

- Augmentation rhinoplasty • Asian rhinoplasty • Alloplast • Silicone • Wing graft

KEY POINTS

- Silicone implants can be safely used for nasal dorsal augmentation if precautions are taken.
- Autologous cartilages are preferred for the tip, in contrast to the dorsum.
- Multiple onlay grafts are stacked to achieve adequate tip projection.
- Septal extension graft provides support and stability for the stacked onlay grafts and prevents deterioration of columellar-lobular ratio.
- The wing grafts are essential to prevent pinching deformity and graft visibility when using multiple onlay grafts.

INTRODUCTION

Dorsal augmentation is a challenging task for rhinoplasty surgeons in Asia because the required amount of augmentation is frequently substantial.

Autologous materials, such as rib cartilages, diced cartilages wrapped in fascia, and dermis or dermofat grafts, are used for dorsal augmentation by many Asian surgeons. However, silicone augmentation is still the dominant practice in Asian countries.

Alloplastic implants have advantages over autologous materials, such as ease of use, unlimited supply of volume, less invasive nature of the procedure, and incomparably superior aesthetic outcomes.

AUGMENTATION RHINOPLASTY USING SILICONE IMPLANTS

Asian rhinoplasty is unique in many aspects. The nasal dorsum of Asians is relatively flat and wide, even though a high and well-defined nasal bridge is preferred in Asian cultures.

There are some aesthetic considerations that need to be comprehended and managed for augmentation rhinoplasty in Asians.

The nose should enhance the beauty of the ethnic Asian face harmonizing with other facial parts, such as relatively flat, rounded forehead and mala. The nose should not stand out too prominently to draw attention from others.

The transition from forehead to nasal bridge is very smooth and gentle, especially in women. The nasofrontal angle in Asians is not structured; rather it is a smooth gracious curvature. When this shallow curvature is obliterated by overaugmentation, an unnatural and operated look will result.

There are some technical difficulties and nuances in Asian rhinoplasty; techniques that are highly successful in Caucasian noses are frequently insufficient or unsatisfactory in Asians.

Small attenuated lower lateral cartilages with short medial crura covered with thick skin make sculpting or suturing tip techniques unsatisfactory in many Asian noses.[1]

Septal extension graft also may not provide sufficient tip projection and definition as desired by the patient. In addition, risk of complications is high, such as septal buckling and tip drooping due to weak caudal septum. Septal cartilages are frequently thin and small, especially in Asian women.

Given that augmentation rhinoplasty is one of the most common aesthetic procedures in Asia, the patient's expectation is generally high on the outcome, and prompt recovery without significant

Disclosure: The author has nothing to disclose.
Doctor Be: Aesthetic Clinic, A238, 316 Eun-ma Shopping Mall, Daechi-Dong, Gangnam-Gu, Seoul 06284, Korea
E-mail address: drbe0911@gmail.com

Facial Plast Surg Clin N Am 26 (2018) 285–293
https://doi.org/10.1016/j.fsc.2018.03.003
1064-7406/18/© 2018 Elsevier Inc. All rights reserved.

morbidity is anticipated. In this regard, silicone is still the material of choice for many surgeons in Asian countries.

Use of rib cartilage is related to chest scarring, possible pneumothorax, prolonged operation time, and high emotional or economic burden on the patient. The rigid immobile tip of rib cartilage is often odd and unpleasing. Also, rib cartilage is not immune to complications. Warping and resorption are frequent, and although infection is uncommon, it is possible. Because of its solid nature it may get fractured with trauma more easily than elastic alloplastic implants. In this regard, rib cartilages are reserved as a last resort rather than as a primary choice for primary aesthetic rhinoplasty by many surgeons. Use of rib cartilage in a primary aesthetic rhinoplasty should be evaluated carefully on the benefits and costs, patient's comfort level, and possibility of overtreatment.

For diced cartilages and dermal/dermofat grafts, inevitable problems exist, for example, resorption, irregularity, insufficient volume, increased operation time, morbidity, and scar in different body parts.

Silicone is free from resorption and deformation. Silicone has advantages over other alloplastic materials as well. Because of its nonporous nature, silicone does not harbor bacteria internally and is easily sterilized with antiseptic solution.[2]

In contrast, porous implants are theoretically more susceptible to infection. Pore size greater than 1 μm allows for ingress of bacteria, whereas macrophages require pore sizes of 30 to 50 μm. Several studies have shown that the risk of infection of biomeshes is influenced by the presence of micropores, as bacteria are able to settle in these structures where they are protected against the actions of macrophages, which cannot penetrate the biomaterial.[3]

Silicone implants are formed from the polymerization of silica (SiO_2) and subsequent crosslinking and extension of the material, which can create either silicone gel or rubber, depending on the specifics of the preparation. Silicone rubber is also available in a range of consistencies, such as soft, medium, and firm.[4]

Silicone rubber resists modification by the host tissue, and it is chemically inert, eliciting only a minimal host response.

Silicone rubber has high resilience against compression or deformation. It maintains its original shape through a wide range of temperatures from $-55°C$ to $+400°C$; therefore, it can be autoclaved without damaging its qualities.[5]

Prefabricated silicone implants are available in different styles in the market; however, they will not correspond to every different style of individual noses. More desirably, each implant is carved for each patient before and during the operation.[6]

The L-shaped silicone implant has been widely used in Asian countries. One of the major advantages of this silicone implant is a smooth and undisrupted nasal dorsal contour from radix to nasal tip. With the L-shaped silicone implant, augmentation of both the nasal dorsum and the tip is accomplished concurrently without complicated tip procedures.

The L-shaped silicone may be an attractive choice for Asian patients because of extreme difficulties of tip plasty in the Asian patient with weak septum, small and weak cartilaginous framework with short medial crura, and thick soft tissue envelope.

However, drawbacks of the L-shaped silicone implant are apparent.

First, risk of tip skin problem, such as extrusion, is high, especially when the implant is excessively long, or the tension on the tip exerted by the implant is high. The implant can extrude through the tip skin or through the membranous septum (**Fig. 1**). Even an implant with a short vertical segment, such as the "bird-shaped" implant, may extrude, because in many cases, those implants are long enough to be in direct contact with the tip skin.

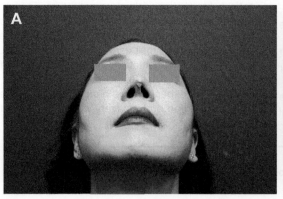 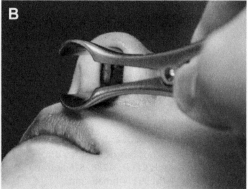

Fig. 1. The implant can extrude through the tip skin or through the membranous septum.

Second, overrotation of the tip is common. With L-silicone, it is very difficult to elongate the tip. Therefore, usually the most projected point of the tip is created in a more rotated position. The consequent infratip lobule is vertically elongated, which is unnatural. This unnatural tip shape is more obvious when it is used for the short nose patient with an overrotated tip.

Third, the resultant tip shape is abnormally narrow and often single pointed. The newly generated tip by the implant is only centrally prominent, which is disharmonious with surrounding wide thick lobules.

Fourth, the "rocker-bottom" phenomenon may arise. With rhinion at the center as a fulcrum, the longer distal part naturally drops inferiorly with time because of gravity, and it is accelerated by gradual resolution of the tension on the tip. As tip projection is lost gradually with the distal implant falling inferiorly, the proximal implant will be lifted, floating on the nasal bone as a consequence, which will create overaugmentation of radix.

Because of these concerns of the L-shaped silicone, the I-shaped silicone implant may be used instead. Using the I-shaped silicone implant, tip augmentation is done separately with autologous cartilages.

For the I-shaped implant, some surgeons are concerned with possible discontinuity between the dorsum and the tip, which may be unapparent until final resolution of postoperative edema.[1]

However, the discontinuity problem can be eliminated by suturing the implant directly to the onlay grafts on the tip, as described later in this article.

Despite potential advantages, use of alloplastic materials in rhinoplasty is often discouraged in Western countries because of concern for possible infection and extrusion of the implant.

In contrast, collective experience of long-term favorable results makes the silicone implants widely used in Asian countries.

Some surgeons suggest that silicone implants are more tolerated by Asians with thick skin; however, it is difficult to stereotype the Asian nasal tip with varying skin thicknesses. Even for thick-skinned patients, excessive tension and irritation or bacterial infection of the implant cannot be tolerated.

Complication rates for silicone implants vary significantly, depending on surgeon's experience, surgical technique, and implant design. Severe complications, in particular, extrusion and infection, are related to faulty techniques rather than the innate property of the material.[7]

Recently reported complication rates have decreased with silicone implants; it may be attributed to improved implant design, use of softer implants, more conservative approach, and better skill and judgment by the surgeon.[8–10]

SURGICAL TECHNIQUES
Draping

Proper draping is important for thorough sterilization of the surgical field. Water-tight draping along the hairline is done using adhesive film drapes clearing hairs out of the field. Nasal vestibular hairs are shaved before draping, and then vestibular skin and anterior nasal cavity are scrubbed carefully with antiseptic-soaked gauzes. Posterior nasal cavity is lightly packed with antiseptic-soaked gauzes also, to decrease aspiration of blood and to decrease the regurgitation of saliva and blood from oral cavity.

Dry gauze or a sanitized mask is gently taped on the upper lip covering the mouth but not obstructing the oral airway.

Implant Design

A correctly designed implant is crucial for a successful outcome.

The thickness of the implant is chosen within the 2- to 10-mm range. Commonly, implants with 2- to 5-mm thickness are selected. For the thickness of the implant, the thinner the better on the premise that the aesthetic value is not compromised too much. The reason why a thinner implant as possible is selected is that when the implant is thicker than 3 mm, although it is variable according to the skin thickness, implant margins may possibly be noticed. However, graft visibility is a common tradeoff for other augmentation materials as well as a tradeoff for autografts.

Depending on the shape of the individual nose, implant design is customized. Initial carving of the implant is done before local anesthetic injection. The implant is carved according to the desired shape of the nose.

For a nose with a low radix and a relatively well-projected tip, the implant is designed thicker in the radix area and gradually thinner approaching the tip area. If a nose has a shallow nasofrontal angle with inadequate tip projection, the implant is made thin on the radix area and gradually thicker on the tip area (**Fig. 2**).

The initially carved implant is applied on the dorsum to examine the general profile of the nose and appropriate length of the implant. The proximal end of the implant is placed at the skin marking, which indicates the nasal starting point usually at the level of the upper ciliary margins. The nasal starting point is assigned variably according to the anatomy of the patient,

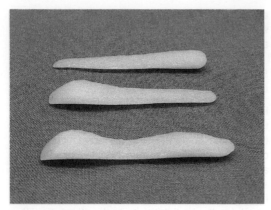

Fig. 2. Implants are designed according to the nasal profile of the patient.

between the supratarsal crease and the midpupillary line.

The proximal implant should not obliterate the nasofrontal angle, but it should blend with the gracious curvature of this region.

During carving, the bottom surface of the implant is carved in a concave shape to match with the convex nasal dorsum. In the rhinion area, more concavity of the implant is frequently required. The lateral and proximal margins of the implant are tapered carefully to prevent implant visibility.

The initially carved implant is preserved in antiseptic solution until further manipulation in later steps.

Incision and Skin Flap Elevation

After local anesthetic injection, a marginal incision is made, and the columellar skin flap is elevated. The skin flap is dissected on the supraperichondrial plane for thin-skinned patients as usual. In contrast, for thick-skinned patients, the skin flap is dissected in the subcutaneous plane for the superficial muscular aponeurotic system debulking or so-called defatting procedure, which is frequently helpful to improve the tip definition. For the defatting procedure, a layer of soft tissue is deliberately left on the surface of the alar cartilages, elevating the skin flap. The thickness of the soft tissue left on the cartilage is varied depending on the thickness of the tip skin. To prevent damage to the dermal plexus of the skin flap during this procedure, a thin fat layer on the undersurface of the skin flap must be preserved. Extensive defatting far laterally or beyond the supra-alar crease should be avoided to preserve proximal blood supply. In the supratip area, the dissection plane is changed to supraperichondrial plane.

Creation of Subperosteal Pocket

It is important to accurately raise the periosteal flap from the nasal bones. Subperiosteal dissection should be limited up to the skin marking of the nasal starting point. More extensive cephalic dissection causes early cephalic migration of the implant and more bleeding from the nasofrontal suture line, which can cause postoperative hematoma.

A vertical line for augmentation along the dorsum, from the nasal tip to the forehead, is marked before draping in a sitting position. Because facial asymmetry is always present to some extent, nasion, rhinion, nasal tip, and philtrum may not be perfectly aligned vertically, and also, bony or cartilage dorsum is frequently asymmetric bilaterally. Therefore, this vertical dorsal line, which looks the straightest for the patient, is helpful for guidance to align the silicone implant, nasal bones, upper and lower lateral cartilages, and tip grafts.

The periosteal flap is elevated first along this vertical dorsal line and is widened bilaterally in a symmetric manner. The size of the subperiosteal pocket is little bit wider, about 10% wider than the width of the implant. If it is too wide, early migration and deviation of the implant will occur. If it is too narrow, however, an unstably or asymmetrically placed implant may also deviate.

Septal Extension Graft

After the defatting procedure is completed, alar cartilages are delineated clearly. Then, membranous septum is dissected to identify the caudal septum, and septal cartilage is harvested. For Asian patients with very weak and thin septal cartilages, the width of the L-strut should be more than the conventional 1 cm for structural stability, even though the available septal cartilage will be smaller.

The septal extension graft is one of the most reliable tip techniques for Asians. It provides a firmer and stronger tip support than the columellar strut.

However, it is frequently insufficient to achieve adequate tip projection required by Asian patients. Overzealous effort to augment the tip using the septal extension graft alone in patients with weak caudal septum frequently results in complications, such as the septal buckling, columellar disfigurement, and long-term drooping of the tip.

Therefore, the tension on the tip by the septal extension graft in these patients should be minimal to moderate, not risking the graft stability.

To prevent complications, the graft should extend posteriorly to overlap the thicker and stronger posterior part of the caudal septum. However, it should not be too deep down to the maxillary crest. If the graft is placed too posteriorly to contact the maxillary crest, there will be no room for graft movement posteriorly, and the chance of tilting or lateral extrusion of the graft is increased as tension is released only laterally. Preservation of a small space between the graft and the maxillary crest for tension release and posterior movement of the graft is desirable. If the graft is placed too anteriorly, however, rotation of graft or septal buckling is complicated as well, because of increased torque on a weaker part of the caudal septum.

For Asian noses, the septal extension graft alone is frequently insufficient, and thus, it is combined with the onlay grafts. When onlay grafts are combined to augment the tip, the septal extension graft has a supportive role rather than the main augmentation method, and the stability of the graft is prioritized over the amount of tip augmentation.

In the combined use with onlay grafts, the septal extension graft also helps to prevent deterioration of columellar-lobular ratio by the multiple onlay grafts.

Temporary Application of the Implant in the Dorsal Pocket

The initially carved implant is positioned inside the dorsal pocket. The nasal profile by the implant is closely examined. Repeated carving and trial of the implant may be necessary until the desired nasal profile is obtained. The implant might be used as a dummy for the tip surgery. The surgeon can estimate the required amount of projection by the implant on the tip, and also the desired amount of rotation/derotation by moving the implant back and forth.

Replacement of the Distal Implant with Stacked Onlay Grafts

To achieve enough tip projection in Asians, stacking of multiple onlay grafts has been advocated.[11,12] Because the available septal cartilage is limited, auricular cartilage is generally used for this purpose.

Usually 2 to 4 layers of auricular cartilages are stacked, as 3 layers of auricular cartilage will be around 5 mm thick. The cephalocaudal length of the stacked graft is little bit longer than that of the domal segment of alar cartilages, and the width is about 7 to 8 mm, corresponding to the natural width of the tip-defining points, which is 6 to 8 mm in women and 8~10 mm in men.

When the stacked onlay grafts are prepared, the same length of the graft is resected from the distal portion of the silicone implant. Then the stacked onlay grafts are sutured to the cut end of the implant.

The stacked onlay grafts are suture-fixated to the implant at the same level or at a slightly higher level of the implant to accentuate the tip projection.

The cut end of the implant may be carved and beveled more to comply with the onlay grafts and inclination of lateral crura of alar cartilages.

The unified graft and implant hybrid are now tried inside the dorsal pocket, and more carving of the implant is done if necessary. When the desired shape of the nose is finally obtained, the onlay grafts are carefully positioned on the tip, and suture-fixated to the caudal margin of alar cartilages (**Fig. 3**).

Usually the dead space in the supratip area between the implant and the dorsum is insignificant for this technique. Careful carving of the implant and use of a soft silicone will minimize the dead space in this area.

However, if a significant dead space is expected because of considerable height difference between the dorsum and the tip, the distal margin of the implant is designed in a wedge shape to fit in the cephalic divergence of the alar cartilages, and the implant is sutured to the lateral crura. Tip augmentation is done separately with onlay or shield grafts (**Fig. 4**).

The Wing Grafts

The most notable drawback of the multiple onlay grafts is the pinched appearance of the nasal tip, which is a result of midline buildup by onlay grafts, with subsequent soft tissue collapse lateral to the onlay grafts.

To prevent the pinching deformity, the wing grafts are applied bilaterally on the lateral sides of the stacked onlay grafts (**Fig. 5**).

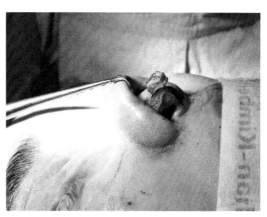

Fig. 3. The onlay grafts are carefully positioned on the tip, and suture-fixated to the caudal margin of alar cartilages.

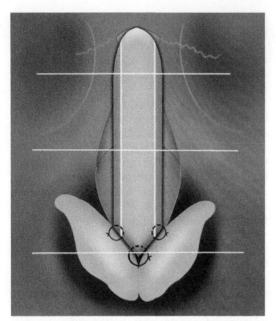

Fig. 4. If a significant dead space is expected because of considerable height difference between the dorsum and the tip, the distal margin of the implant is designed in a wedge shape to fit in the cephalic divergence of the alar cartilages, and the implant is sutured to the lateral crura.

They provide structural support for alar lobules and alar rims against soft tissue collapse; and they provide smooth undisrupted transition of contour from the tip to the alar lobules and efface the margins of the onlay grafts decreasing the graft visibility. They act as new lateral crura corresponding to the newly created dome by the onlay grafts.

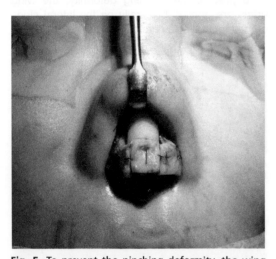

Fig. 5. To prevent the pinching deformity, the wing grafts are applied bilaterally on the lateral sides of the stacked onlay grafts to prevent the pinching deformity.

Auricular cartilages are best suited for this purpose because of their natural curvature.

The size and inclination of the wing grafts can be varied according to the intention of surgery.

The wing grafts also can be used to treat the alar rim retraction. Because they are securely fixed to the onlay grafts medially like the articulated rim grafts, they provide stronger support against retraction comparing with the alar rim grafts.

The final fine modification of the tip shape is achieved by delicate carving of the onlay grafts and application of additional shield or onlay grafts as necessary.

This technique, which combines the stacked onlay grafts with the septal extension graft, is very effective for elongation of the tip as necessary, and amount of tip augmentation is almost unrestricted (**Fig. 6**).

A representative case is shown in **Fig. 7**.

In contrast, for the widely used techniques using silicone implants, the tip of the silicone implant (straight or L-shaped) is placed on top of the dome, and a piece of autologous cartilage is laid on top or in front of the distal implant to prevent

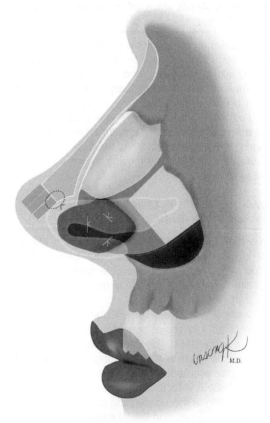

Fig. 6. Combining the stacked onlay grafts with the septal extension graft is very effective for elongation of the tip and tip augmentation.

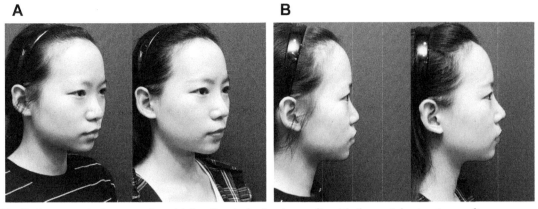

Fig. 7. A representative case of combining the stacked onlay grafts with the septal extension graft.

skin problems. These techniques readily provide tip projection and rotation with the silicone implant and produce fair outcomes in selected cases, especially in those with underrotated nasal tips. However, these techniques tend to create an over-rotated and unnatural nasal tip. Tip projection and rotation increase without proportional elongation of the tip. The infratip lobule is vertically elongated and unnatural with a decreased columellar-lobular ratio. The tip is often only centrally prominent with varying degrees of pinched appearance. Fine tip modification is also difficult in these techniques.

COMPLICATIONS

Some complications related to silicone implants are serious, requiring immediate and decisive management, and some complications are less serious and can be treated with less aggressive maneuvers.

Serious complications are infection, implant extrusion, and severe capsular contracture. Less serious complications are deviation, visibility, calcification, and others. Serious complications are very rare in experienced hands, and related more to technical errors by the surgeon rather than the inherent traits of silicone material, as discussed later. Fortunately, serious complications are avoidable and can be reduced.

Infection

Infection is the most dreaded and troublesome complication, which must be avoided with meticulous preventive measures.

Alloplastic implants are susceptible to infection and, when infected, exhibit typical symptoms, such as erythema, swelling, and purulent discharge.

Delayed infection is also possible, and it is often subtle and less obvious, presenting as late recurrent swelling or mild erythema. There is evidence

that chronic indolent but relapsing infection is related to bacterial biofilm on the surface of the implant.[13–15]

Bacterial biofilm causes infection and inflammation of indolent nature in which traditional culture fails to recover any isolates.

To prevent bacterial contamination, thorough sterilization of the surgical field is important. During surgery, frequent scrubbing of gloves and instruments with antiseptic solution is mandated. The implant is immersed in sterilizing solution between procedures. It is important to prevent disruption of natural barriers, such as mucous membrane, during surgery. Osteotomies are not an absolute contraindication for silicone augmentation; however, the surgeon should be very careful to minimize mucosal tearing during osteotomies and humpectomies.

A lengthy surgical time is related to decreased blood flow to the soft tissue and more chance of infection; therefore, the surgeon should try to reduce the surgical time as much as possible.

Extrusion

Reported extrusion rates of silicone implants vary from 0.48% to 50%, probably due to the differences in surgical technique, implant shape, and the surgeon's level of experience.[8,16,17]

Roughly, there are 2 sources of the problem. One is a poorly designed implant with excessive length, and the other source is infection. An excessively long implant may extrude through the tip skin or into the nasal cavity. A poorly designed implant, which is not stabilized in the nasofrontal angle or in the subperiosteal pocket, may migrate distally.

Excessive pressure exerted by the L-silicone on the tip is associated with higher risk of extrusion. Extrusion is often caused by infection. An implant may extrude through inflamed and macerated soft tissue with a variable degree of purulence.

Sometimes, infection is less obvious with only minimal granulation tissue surrounding the implant. In such cases, the surgeon should be aware of the possibility of infection.

Capsular Contracture

Capsule formation is a natural host reaction to silicone implants. Fibrous capsule protects the skin and surrounding tissue isolating the implant. However capsular contracture is serious in some cases. Infection is the most well-known cause of serious capsular contracture. Severe capsular contracture often occurs after apparent infection or after removal of an infected implant.

There are multiple clinical studies that have demonstrated significant correlation between presence of biofilms/bacterial colonization and capsular contracture of breast implants.[18]

An abnormally thick capsule will accompany varying degrees of contracture, which is related to various factors as well as infection, biofilm, such as nonimplantable or even nonmedical grade silicones, excessive soft tissue damage by overly aggressive techniques, and chronic inflammation or irritation by micromovement of the implant.

Capsular contracture is a frequent problem for silicone breast implants as well. Normally, severe capsular contracture of breast implants is reduced by antibiotic irrigation, antifibroblastic medications, and elimination of aggravating factors, such as soft tissue damage and intraoperative bleeding. These preventive measures and techniques may be applied to nasal implants.

Minor Complications

There are less serious complications, such as calcification, deviation, implant movability, and displacement.

Calcification is more common in silicone implants than in porous implants. It is more frequent for long-seated implants and may worsen with time. However, it is also influenced by technical factors, such as chronic mechanical stimulation of soft tissue by poorly designed movable implants and intraoperative damage to surrounding soft tissue.[19] Use of a softer implant, decreasing implant movability, and decrease of soft tissue damage during operation may reduce calcification.

Deviation, movability, and displacement issues are avoided by proper implant design, adequate dorsal pocket formation, implant fixation, and nasal splinting after surgery. Careful implant placement in a properly created subperiosteal pocket as opposed to the subfascial or subcutaneous space reduces implant mobility and may decrease risk of displacement.[2]

SUMMARY

Complication rates for silicone implants vary significantly, depending on surgeon's experience, surgical technique, and implant design. Severe complications, such as extrusion and infection, are rare, and they are more commonly related to faulty techniques rather than inherent characteristics of the material. Silicone implants can be safely used for nasal dorsal augmentation if precautions are taken as carefully outlined in this article.

In contrast to the dorsum, for the tip augmentation, autologous cartilages are preferred.

Because the required amount of the tip augmentation is frequently substantial for Asians, stacked onlay grafts combined with the septal extension graft are used for the tip augmentation. The wing grafts are essential to prevent graft visibility and pinching deformity in using the stacked onlay grafts.

REFERENCES

1. McCurdy JA. The Asian nose: augmentation rhinoplasty with L-shaped silicone implants. Facial Plast Surg 2002;18(4):245–52.
2. Genther DJ, Papel ID. Surgical nasal implants: indications and risks. Facial Plast Surg 2016;32:488–99.
3. Perez-Köhler B, Bayon Y, Bellon JM. Mesh infection and hernia repair: a review. Surg Infect (Larchmt) 2016;20(10):1–14.
4. Ferril GR, Wudel JM, Winkler AA. Management of complications from alloplastic implants in rhinoplasty. Facial Plast Surg 2013;4(21):372–8.
5. Colas A, Curtis J. Medical applications of silicones. Biomaterials science. 2nd edition. New York: Elsevier Inc; 2004. p. 697–707.
6. Erlich MA, Parhiscar A. Nasal dorsal augmentation with silicone implants. Facial Plast Surg 2003;19:325–30.
7. McCurdy JA, Lam SM. Cosmetic surgery of the Asian face. London: Thieme Medical Publishers; 2005.
8. Peled ZM, Warren AG, Johnston P, et al. The use of alloplastic materials in rhinoplasty surgery: a meta-analysis. Plast Reconstr Surg 2008;121(3):85e–92e.
9. Lam SM, Kim YK. Augmentation rhinoplasty of the Asian nose with the "bird" silicone implant. Ann Plast Surg 2003;51:249–56.
10. Tham C, Lai YL, Weng CJ, et al. Silicone augmentation rhinoplasty in an Oriental population. Ann Plast Surg 2005;54:1–5.
11. Ahn J, Horando C, Horn C. Combined silicone and cartilage implants: augmentation rhinoplasty in

Asian patients. Arch Facial Plast Surg 2004;6(2): 120–3.

12. Jang YJ, Hong HR. Augmentation shield grafts. JAMA Facial Plast Surg 2015;17(4):301–2.

13. Tamboto H, Vickery K, Sc MV, et al. Subclinical (biofilm) infection causes capsular contracture in a procine model following augmentation mammoplasty. Plast Reconstr Surg 2010;126:835–42.

14. Mohan K, Cox JA, Dickey RM, et al. Treatment of infected facial implants. Semin Plast Surg 2016;30: 78–82.

15. Walker TJ, Toriumi DM. Analysis of facial implants for bacterial biofilm formation using scanning electron microscopy. JAMA Facial Plast Surg 2016;18(4): 299–304.

16. Lee MR, Unger JG, Rohrich RJ. Management of the nasal dorsum in rhinoplasty: a systemic review of the literature regarding technique, outcomes, and complications. Plast Reconstr Surg 2011;128:538e–50e.

17. Loyo M, Ishii LE. Safety of alloplastic materials in rhinoplasty. JAMA Facial Plast Surg 2013;15:162–3.

18. Ajdic D, Zoghbi Y, Gerth D, et al. The relationship of bacterial biofilms and capsular contracture in breast implants. Aesthet Surg J 2016;36(3):297–309.

19. Jung DH, Kim BR, Rho YS, et al. Gross and pathologic analysis of long-term silicone implants inserted into the human body for augmentation rhinoplasty: 221 revision cases. Plast Reconstr Surg 2007;120: 1997–2003.

Dorsal Augmentation Using Autogenous Tissues

Man-Koon Suh, MD*

KEYWORDS

- Asian rhinoplasty • Dorsal augmentation • Diced cartilage • Dermofat graft • Temporal fascia
- Costal cartilage graft • Folded dermal graft

KEY POINTS

- Autogenous tissues used for major dorsal augmentation in Asian noses are dermofat, solid block costal cartilage, and diced cartilage.
- Vertically oriented folded dermal graft technique provides high profile graft, minimizes resorption, and is a good technique for major dorsal augmentation.
- A solid block costal cartilage graft permits the largest amount of dorsal augmentation among autogenous tissues, and provides more defined dorsum.
- The diced cartilage graft shows less resorption than dermofat graft, and can be easily performed by novice surgeons.

Unlike Western nations, the material most commonly used for dorsal augmentation in Asian countries still is an implant. The reason is that an implant not only provides a further defined and more beautiful dorsal shape, but also requires shorter operating time without the donor site morbidity associated with autogenous tissue harvesting. Nonetheless, nasal dorsal augmentation using autogenous tissue still is the ultimate goal for aesthetic rhinoplastic surgeons, because autogenous tissue is less likely to cause implant-related complications such as infection, dorsal skin thinning and redness, capsular contracture, and implant exposure through the tip skin or vestibular mucosa. Autogenous tissues used for major dorsal augmentation of Asians are largely dermofat, solid block type costal cartilage, and diced cartilage.

DORSAL AUGMENTATION WITH DERMOFAT

Dermofat graft is the most commonly used autogenous tissue for dorsal augmentation in East Asian countries.[1] In particular, dermofat graft can be most safely performed to the thinned dorsal skin after the removal of illegally injected foreign liquid material to the dorsum, which was rather common in some Asian countries.[2]

Operative Technique

Harvest procedures

In the sacrococcygeal area, the dermis is thicker than anywhere else in the body. In addition, the subdermal fat layer is relatively dense. These anatomic properties of the sacrococcygeal soft tissue create for an excellent source of dermofat graft.[3] This is also one of the most covered areas of the body, and postoperative scars are inconspicuous. A graft is harvested from 1 side of the buttock close to the intergluteal crease. The medial margin of the graft is located about 2 to 3 mm lateral to the crease (**Fig. 1**). The dermofat will undergo contracture immediately upon harvest. Thus, the design of dermofat should incorporate larger-than-needed dimensions to account for the contracture. For the purpose of dorsal augmentation, the author

Disclosure: The author has nothing to disclose.
JW Plastic Surgery Center, Seoul, Republic of Korea
* 3rd Floor, Samshin Building, Shinsa dong, Gangnam gu, Seoul 135-893, Republic of Korea.
E-mail address: smankoon@hanmail.net

Facial Plast Surg Clin N Am 26 (2018) 295–310
https://doi.org/10.1016/j.fsc.2018.03.004
1064-7406/18/© 2018 Elsevier Inc. All rights reserved.

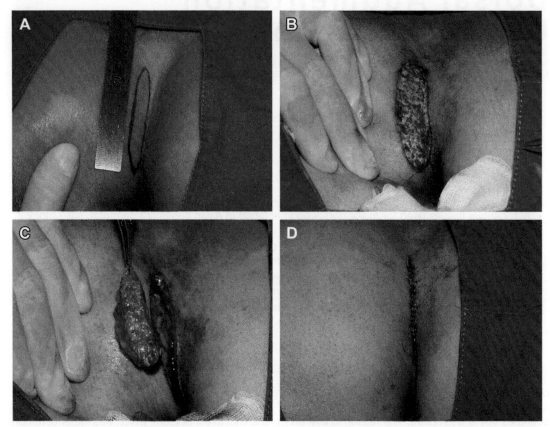

Fig. 1. Harvesting the dermofat graft. (*A*) Graft is harvested from one side of the buttock close to the intergluteal crease. (*B*) After the skin incision along the designed line, deepithelization is performed. (*C*) The dermis and fat layer are harvested. (*D*) Wound closure.

harvests dermofat that is 60 mm long, 10 to 12 mm wide, and 6 to 10 mm deep. The author designs the lowermost point of the incision at least 3 cm above the anus.

The skin is incised using a No. 15 blade without exposing the subcutaneous fat. The dermis is deepithelized by peeling off the epidermis using a No. 10 blade. Incomplete removal of epidermis should be avoided because it can result in epidermal cyst at the graft site. Upon complete deepithelizaiton, the dermal incision is carried down into the subcutaneous tissue. Once the incision is at an adequate depth, the whole graft is elevated en bloc.

Dorsal augmentation technique

Unlike silicone implants, dermofat grafts are placed in the supraperichondrial and supraperiosteal planes.

The superior end of a silicone implant is usually placed at the height of upper eyelash line or the supratarsal fold. The dermofat graft should be placed a bit more cephalically than this upper point. For most patients, the author finds the

midpoint between the supratarsal crease and the eyebrow to be appropriate (**Fig. 2**). This placement will tend to result in a natural augmentation of the radix upon partial resorption of the dermofat. Inferiorly, the caudal endpoint of dermofat should reach to the nasal tip.

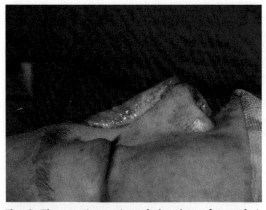

Fig. 2. The starting point of the dermofat graft is approximately the midpoint between the double eyelid crease and eyebrow.

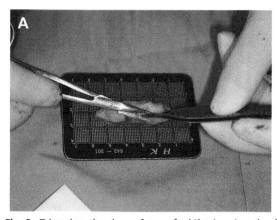
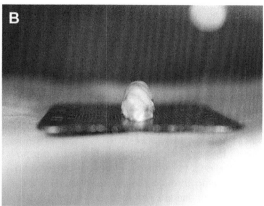

Fig. 3. Trimming the dermofat graft. (*A*) trimming the fat portion of the graft. (*B*) The graft's shape resembles that of the implant, whose roof side is narrower than the bottom side.

Before insertion, the dermofat should be trimmed to appropriate width and shape. Usually, a graft width of 10 mm is appropriate, but this should be tailored to the width of each individual nose. Akin to the shape of silicone implants, the dermofat should be contoured such that the floor is wider and the roof is narrower (**Fig. 3**). Regarding the orientation of dermofat, the conventional practice is to place the dermis side up and subcutaneous down within the graft pocket, the idea being that the proximity of the deepithelized dermis to the nasal skin allowing neovascularization and increasing graft survival.[4] In practice, however, this author thinks that the orientation of dermofat placement does not affect the resorption of the graft so much. Additionally, placing the graft such that the fat layer is on top facilitates the shaping the graft more easily. For fixation, the cephalic end of dermofat graft is secured using a pull-out suture between the eyebrows. The caudal end of the graft is fixed to the septal angle or the dome of lower lateral cartilage using a 5-0 polydioxanone suture (**Fig. 4**). The pull-out suture is removed a week after the operation.

The dermofat graft can undergo partial resorption up to 18 months after the operation. The resorption rate increases with the amount of fat tissue. Some authors reported as much as 70% resorption rate.[5] Other authors reported that 25% to 30% overcorrection would be sufficient, but an approximately 40% to 60% or higher resorption rate is generally considered to be average. Thus, overcorrection should be performed in consideration of this resorption rate. Surgeons must also consider the patient's psychological uneasiness toward unnatural height and shape, secondary to overcorrection, in the early postoperative period. Therefore, an overcorrection of 30% to 40% is usually appropriate. However, resorption rates vary widely across

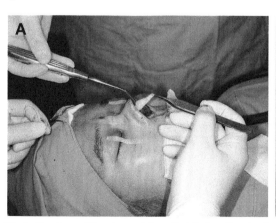
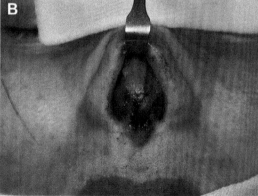

Fig. 4. Fixation of the dermofat graft. (*A*) A pull-out suture is used to fix the cephalic end of the graft to the area between the eye brows. (*B*) The caudal end of the graft is fixed to the septal angle or dome of the lower lateral cartilage.

individuals and cannot be predicted in an accurate manner.

Resorption occurs until approximately 16 months after surgery, but there is not much change thereafter (**Fig. 5**). In most cases, an unsatisfactory dorsal height is shown owing to the high absorption rate, necessitating an additional procedure such as fat injection.

Indications for dermofat graft

Despite the relatively high resorption rate, dermofat graft allows for a natural dorsal augmentation. Graft showing through the dorsal skin, skin thinning, and redness are not noticed. Therefore, dermofat graft is appropriate for the following situations.

1. Patients with very thin dorsal skin of nose in whom silicone implants may become conspicuous or cause dorsal skin redness.

2. Patients who are apprehensive about silicone or Goretex implant.
3. Secondary rhinoplasty for skin thinning or redness from implant material.
4. After removal of injected materials (eg, liquid silicone), the dorsal skin may be extremely thin with an irregular texture. In such cases, implants or cartilage grafts can show through the thin skin, and dermofat graft would be more appropriate.
5. Correction of minor depression or irregularity in the dorsum, ala, or tip.

Vertically Oriented Folded Dermal Graft Technique

Dermofat graft undergoes resorption in both dermal layer and fat layer, but this resorption is greater in the fat layer. To retain the maximum amount of dorsal augmentation, the thickness of

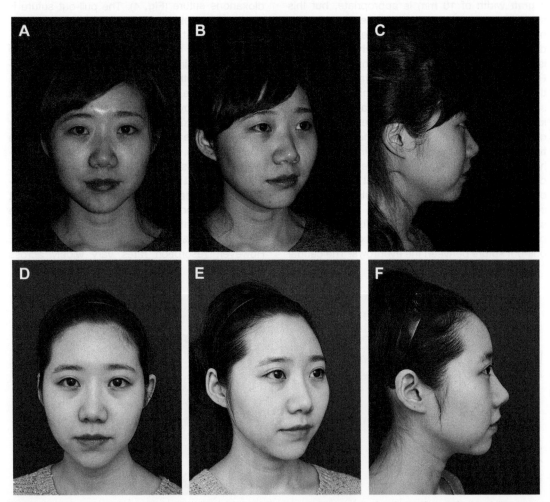

Fig. 5. Preoperative and postoperative views of dorsal augmentation using the dermofat graft. (*A–C*) Preoperative view. (*D–F*) Three years after dermofat graft for the low dorsum and conchal cartilage onlay graft for the tip projection.

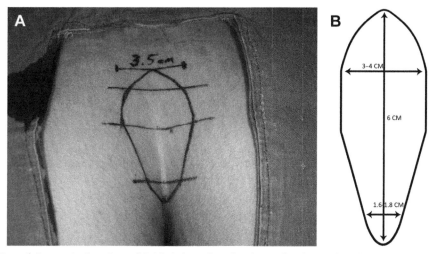

Fig. 6. Design of the vertically oriented folded dermal graft. The graft is located at the midline of the sacrococcygeal area, and the caudal end of the graft is located 2 cm above the coccyx. The length of the graft is 6 cm, the width of the cephalic area is 3 to 4 cm, and that of the caudal area is 1.6 to 1.8 cm.

dermal layer should be maximized, while minimizing the thickness of the fat layer. Some authors reported dermal graft for dorsal augmentation.[6,7] Nevertheless, there are difficulties in the correction of very low dorsum of Asians, owing to limitations in human dermal thickness. Kim and Rhee[8] reported dorsal augmentation using folded dermal graft. However, the technique, which enables

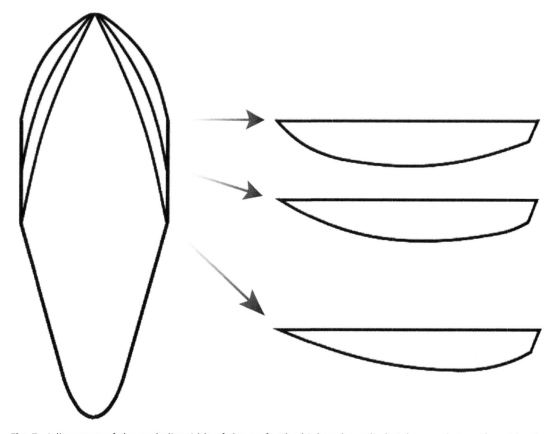

Fig. 7. Adjustment of the cephalic width of the graft. The higher the radix height one desires, the wider the width of the cephalic area of the graft should be designed.

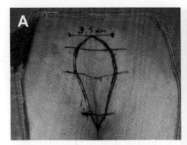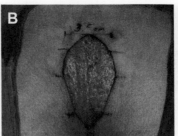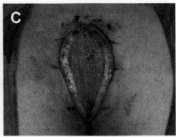

Fig. 8. Harvest of the vertically oriented folded dermal graft. (*A*) An incision is made along the incision line into the half-thickness depth of the dermis. (*B*) The epidermal layer has been peeled off from the dermal layer. (*C*) A deeper dermis incision is made to reach a part of subcutaneous fat layer.

much higher dorsal augmentation, is a vertically oriented folded dermal graft technique that was first presented by Cho.[9]

Design on the donor site

With the patient in prone position, the graft is designed in the sacrococcygeal area as shown in **Fig. 6**. The inferior endpoint of graft is located 2 cm superior to the coccyx. The superior portion

of the graft design can be altered depending on how much of the radix is to be raised (**Fig. 7**). The cephalic portion of the graft needs to be wider for greater augmentation of the radix area.

Harvest of the graft

The graft harvest begins with incision through half the thickness of dermis as seen in **Fig. 8**. Then, deepthelization is performed. Thereafter, the

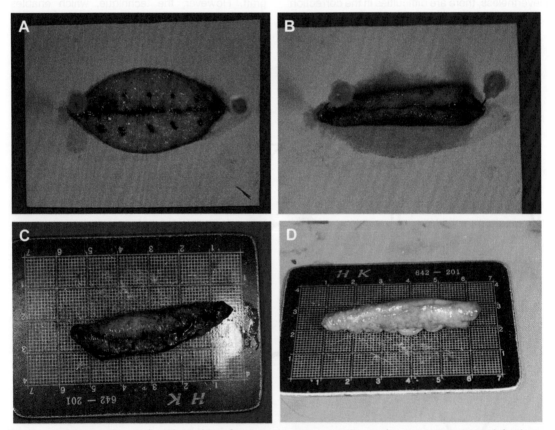

Fig. 9. Fabrication of a graft. (*A*) Marking for 5 inner sutures to the graft containing minimal fat layer, (*B*) Five inner sutures were placed using a No. 6-0 nylon suture. (*C*) The graft base was trimmed to remove the bulging after outer horizontal sutures. (*D*) The graft is erected in a vertical orientation after all the sutures have been placed.

incision is carried into the subcutaneous fat layer. The graft is elevated while incorporating a minimal amount of the fat into the graft.

Wound closure

The donor site should be closed without undermining the skin to minimize the risk of necrosis in the wound margin. The dermal layer is closed using no. 3-0 suture Vicryl sutures, and the skin is closed using no. 3-0 nylon sutures. Drains are not necessary.

Fabrication of the harvested graft

The graft fabrication uses multiple sutures to fold the graft such that it becomes more compact horizontally and provides maximal height. The harvested graft is fixated to a thick paper plate with a pin on each end. A portion of the subcutaneous

fat is trimmed to leave a minimal amount of fat, such that the combined thickness of the dermis and fat ends up around 4 mm (**Fig. 9**). A straight line is drawn along the central axis of the graft, with 2 offset lines on either side. The graft is folded in half along the central line by placing five 6-0 nylon sutures through the offset lines. The folded edges are brought together in 4 places using 5-0 nylon sutures, and this becomes the graft base. Next, the graft is made more compact by the use of multiple outer vertical or horizontal sutures (5-0 nylon). If bulging of the graft's base occurs owing to these sutures, the base is trimmed until it is flat. Next, the outer circular sutures are placed using 5-0 nylon. At this point, the graft should stand vertically on its base as shown in **Fig. 9**. The final height of the fabricated graft should be around 10 to 12 mm.

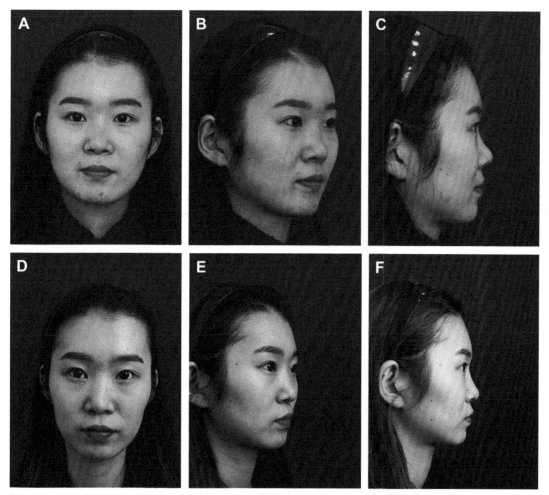

Fig. 10. Case with a vertically oriented folded dermal graft for dorsal augmentation. (*A–C*) Preoperative views. (*D–F*) One year after dorsal augmentation surgery using a vertically oriented folded dermal graft and tip plasty with a derotation suture and conchal cartilage shield graft.

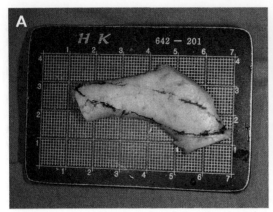
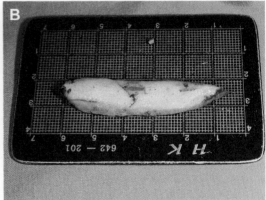

Fig. 11. Concentric carving of the costal cartilage to minimize the graft warping.

Placing the graft on the dorsum

The cephalic end of the graft is fixated to the radix using a pull-out suture. The caudal end is fixed to the septal angle or to the dome of lower lateral cartilages.

Pearls and pitfalls

The vertically oriented folded dermal graft augments the dorsal height not by the thickness, but rather by the folded height of the graft and is conceptually distinct from simple dermofat graft. Because of this, the graft base should be flat enough not to fall to the side when placed on top of the dorsum to prevent deviation of the graft.

An additional matter of importance is to make the graft's width narrow and compact by the use of multiple sutures.

Folded dermal grafts are known to have resorption rates of 40% after 1 year.[8] The absorption rate for the vertically oriented folded dermal graft has not been reported yet (**Fig. 10**).

DORSAL AUGMENTATION WITH SOLID BLOCK COSTAL CARTILAGE

Costal cartilages are abundant in graft volume, and the absorption rate is very low in comparison with the dermofat graft, having the advantage of providing significant augmentation to nasal dorsum. Nonetheless, donor site morbidities such as pneumothorax and chest wall scar are possible in harvesting the costal cartilage,[10] and a highly masterful skill is required in carving and placing the graft. However, an elaborate skill performed by an experienced surgeon can yield much better, well-defined, predictable shape compared with dermofat or diced cartilage. This author believes that the solid block costal cartilage can be an excellent choice for Asians with a very low dorsum,

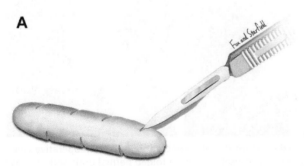
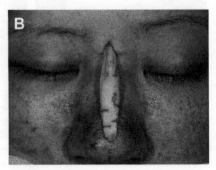

Fig. 12. Multiple full-thickness cuttings on the both margins of the graft can control the warping to some degree.

requiring major dorsal augmentation of 5 mm or more.

Harvest of the Costal Cartilage

Compared with the graft harvested for septal extension graft, the costal cartilage needed for dorsal augmentation needs to be longer—around 5 to 6 cm. Because the seventh rib is relatively longer and straight, the seventh rib cartilage is usually preferable for the purpose of dorsal augmentation.[11] Because the seventh rib is often inaccessible from the inframammary fold, the incision is usually made directly over the seventh rib cartilage to be harvested.

Carving the Costal Cartilage

Carving of the costal cartilage is the most important, difficult, and time-consuming step for successful dorsal augmentation. A graft must be precisely carved to fit to the dorsal shape. If the operator is unable to carve the graft to the requisite dimensions and shape (width, bottom contour, and slope/convexity of both side walls), the graft will not maintain an accurate and even contact surface with the radix and dorsum, and can develop graft deviation or visible graft margins.

The total thickness of harvested costal cartilage must be used for dorsal augmentation in most Asian patients with a very low dorsum. Respecting the principle of balanced cross-section, one can minimize graft warping by the concentric carving of the core cartilage (**Fig. 11**). A thick solid costal cartilage graft that is carved following this principle for dorsal augmentation is fairly resistant to warping. As such, the author avoids the use of K-wire technique reported by Gunter and colleagues,[12]

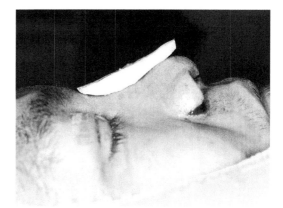

Fig. 14. The graft must be carved to fit in anatomically to the contour of the dorsum and particularly the radix area of the patient.

with which a K-wire is inserted into the center of the costal cartilage.

The graft is designed with the core cartilage as the graft center. The silicone implant that best matches the desired profile is placed on the dorsum of the patient, and the cartilage block is carved to match the shape of this implant as much as possible. First, the periphery of designed graft is trimmed using a No. 10 blade. The resulting block is further shaped using the scalpel and electric burr to match the width and concavity of the nasal dorsum. A graft to be placed in the radix and supratip is carved narrower than that to be placed in the midvault. It is important that the bottom surface of graft accurately matches the dorsal alignment. The cephalic portion of the graft must be carved to fit in with the radix

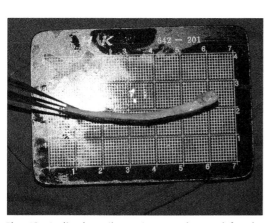

Fig. 13. A sliced cartilage piece can be used for the small amount of dorsal augmentation.

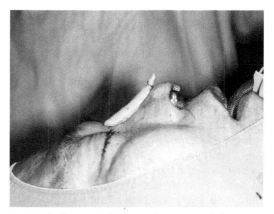

Fig. 15. In the event the smooth contour of the supratip break area cannot be created, 2 pieces of the costal cartilage may be connected to make the supratip break.

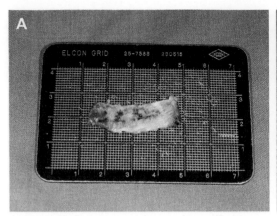
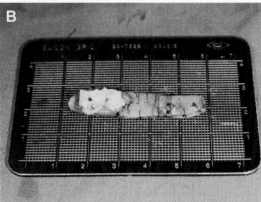

Fig. 16. Perichondrial fixation method. The costal perichondrium is sutured to the undersurface of the graft.

alignment, which would be the most demanding process. If necessary, the cephalic portion of the graft can be made to bend by applying several back-cuts on the bottom of the cephalic portion of the graft.

A carved costal cartilage will have undergone the maximum amount of warping after an hour. As such, the carved graft should be placed in a saline solution for an hour, after which the graft should be further trimmed before insertion. Excessive warping can be adjusted by the placement of several full-thickness cuts on both sides of the graft. This process requires a significant experience (**Fig. 12**). Noses requiring a lesser amount of dorsal augmentation are corrected with implantation of one thin slice of costal cartilage after slicing the harvested costal cartilage into 3 to 4 pieces of appropriate thickness (**Fig. 13**). The concave side of a warped piece is placed toward the dorsum to avoid the graft protruding in the radix and supratip areas.[11] Somewhat excessive warping can be overcome by (1) scoring the concave side of the warped graft, (2) making a horizontal double mattress suture, (3) placing anther small cartilage piece with a curvature of the opposite side, and (4) making a suture fixation of the graft over the underlying upper lateral cartilage. The costal cartilage has a relatively slippery texture and can be easily deviated from its initial position. Therefore, it is very important to carve the cartilage in a meticulous manner such that the resulting graft has an anatomically exact contour to maximize the contact surface between graft and nasal dorsum (**Fig. 14**). This technique not only prevents graft dislocation but also minimizes the risk of infection by decreasing the dead space beneath the graft.

Two graft pieces can be joined together to create the natural curvature of supratip break (**Fig. 15**).

Placement of the Graft on the Dorsum

To prevent the graft deviation, the follow key points should be respected.

1. The size of the subperiosteal pocket, into which the graft is placed, should not be wide. The graft should fit into the pocket tightly to minimize graft movement.
2. Toriumi[11,13–15] suggested the "perichondrial fixation method," using a costal cartilage dorsal graft and interpositional costal perichondrial graft (**Fig. 16**). According to his technique, a

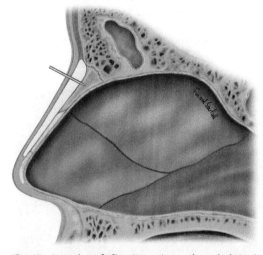

Fig. 17. Dorsal graft fixation using a threaded K-wire. After making a stab incision in the radix skin, a K-wire is passed through the graft and underlying nasal bone. The K-wire is cut, leaving 10 mm above the area of skin incision.

strip of costal perichondrium is sutured to the undersurface of the upper third of the dorsal graft to create a costal/perichondrial interface. Then multiple holes are made in the bony dorsum of the nose using a 2-mm straight osteotome or a narrow rasp is used to create a rough surface on the bony dorsum. And then, the dorsal graft with intervening costal/perichondrial graft is placed on top of the bony dorsum. The raw surface of the bony dorsum and intervening costal perichondrium, together with the tight subperiosteal pocket, prevents slippage, movement, or deviation of the graft.
3. The graft is fixed to the upper lateral cartilage using 5-0 polydioxanone sutures. Two sutures should be placed to the cephalic and caudal portions of the upper lateral cartilage.

4. Threaded K-wire fixations are reserved for special cases where the graft movement cannot be restricted owing to loose periosteum, or in secondary rhinoplasty cases where a narrow pocket cannot be formed.[16] The K-wire is driven through the skin, graft, and underlying nasal bone, to be removed a week after the operation (**Fig. 17**).

On the thin-skinned nose, a diced cartilage is packed loosely along the bilateral margins of the block costal graft and molded to avoid any lateral step-off. Temporal fascia or crushed costal perichondrium of the costal cartilage can be used alternatively. **Figs. 18** and **19** show the examples of dorsal augmentation using a solid block costal cartilage graft.

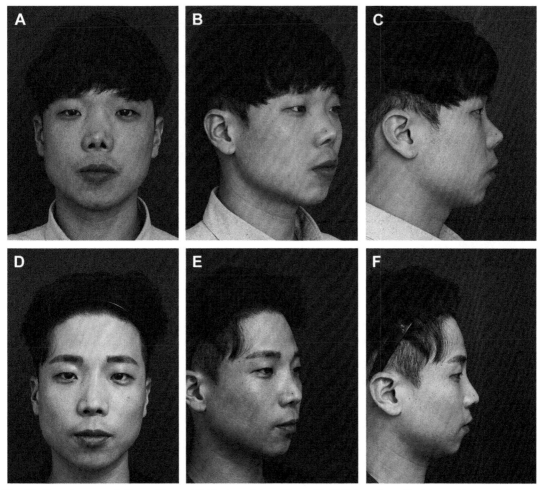

Fig. 18. Dorsal augmentation with a solid block costal cartilage. (*A–C*) This male patient has a flat nasal dorsum, upturned tip, and retracted ala of the left side owing to contracture after removal of the exposed silicone implant through the vestibular mucosa. (*D–F*) Eight months after surgery (dorsal augmentation using solid block costal cartilage graft with 6 mm in height and tip revisional surgery with derotation graft using the auricular cartilage).

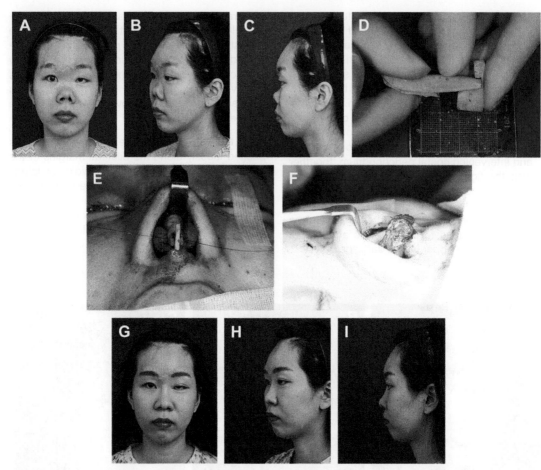

Fig. 19. Dorsal augmentation with 2 layered solid block costal cartilages. (*A–C*) After a traffic accident, this female patient has a saddle nose, collapsed nasal bone, and upturned nasal tip. (*D*) Two layered carved costal cartilage is ready for dorsal augmentation of about 10 mm in height. A small piece of the costal cartilage is attached to the caudal end of the dorsal graft as a tongue-in-groove pattern to lengthen the upturned nasal tip. (*E*) The graft is placed in position. (*F*) Lower lateral cartilages are sutured to the end of the graft. (*G–I*) Two years after surgery.

DORSAL AUGMENTATION WITH DICED CARTILAGE WRAPPED IN TEMPORAL FASCIA

The most highly recommended cartilage graft for major dorsal augmentation in Asian patients is the costal cartilage, because it provides enough volume of cartilaginous material needed to augment the low dorsum. Nevertheless, warping and grafts showing through the thin skin are the major disadvantage of a solid block costal cartilage graft.[17,18] Another technique to overcome such drawbacks is diced cartilage wrapped in temporal fascia (**Fig. 20**).

The use of a diced cartilage graft had been reported decades ago, but was supplanted by the introduction of silicone implants. In 2000, Erol[19] reported a new technique of dorsal augmentation using diced cartilage wrapped in Surgicell—the "Turkish delight" —which again brought the diced cartilage into contemporary practice. Unlike the original report, however, Daniel and colleagues[16,20] found that the graft undergoes total resorption and suggested foreign body reaction against Surgicell as the cause. Thus, they reported a modified technique called diced cartilage wrapped in temporal fascia. The method has been readily adopted by numerous surgeons owing to easy surgical procedure and reduced resorption rate. Diced cartilage grafting is a very useful technique for smoothing out dorsal irregularities or dorsal augmentation.

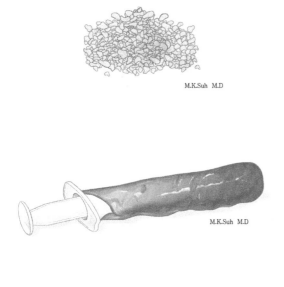

M.K.Suh M.D

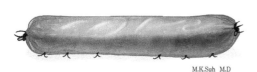

M.K.Suh M.D

Fig. 20. Diced cartilage wrapped in temporal fascia.

Free diced cartilage is used for minor dorsal augmentation, correction of dorsal irregularity, and lateral stepoff after block costal cartilage graft.[21,22] For major dorsal augmentation, it is preferable to use diced cartilage wrapped in temporal fascia.

Harvest of Temporal Fascia

The deep temporal fascia is harvested in a rectangular shape, about 5 × 3 cm. For thin-skinned nasal dorsum, a larger fascia can be harvested such that the overlapping portion of the wrapped fascia is oriented toward the skin, such that there is an extra layer of fascia tissue between the skin and diced cartilage pieces. This technique helps to minimize the risk of irregular texture.

Packing the Diced Cartilage in the Tube-Shaped Fascia

All types of cartilage (conchal, septum, costal) are diced into small pieces of less 0.2 mm in diameter, using a No. 11 or dermatome blade. Costal cartilage is the preferable source when a great quantity of cartilage is required for very low dorsum of

Asians. The diced cartilage is packed into a 1-mL insulin syringe, and the hub of syringe is cut off using a No. 10 blade.

On a plate, the harvested fascia is laid flat, upon which the syringe is placed. The fascia is wrapped around the syringe, and the longitudinal margins of the fascia are closed by continuous running suture using an absorbable suture. The distal end of the fascia is also closed with an absorbable suture. Then the flat fascia turns into a tube around the syringe (**Fig. 21**).

The diced cartilage within the syringe is slowly and gently injected into the fascial tube. While palpating for cartilage particles filling up, the syringe is slowly withdrawn from the tube. The amount of diced cartilage to be filled into the fascia depends on the amount of augmentation desired. After completing the infusion of the cartilage particles, the fascial sleeve on the opposite side is also sutured with an absorbable suture, closing the fascia tube.

If the dorsum needs to be augmented by a large amount of diced cartilage, as much as a 3 to 4 mL or more, a 3-mL syringe, instead of a 1-mL insulin syringe, is used to be wrapped by the fascia.

Insertion of the Diced Cartilage in Fascia to the Pocket

The pocket is placed in the supraperichondrial and subperiosteal plane, and the pocket should be slightly wider than the graft itself. The cephalic end of the graft is fixed with a pull-out suture, and the distal end is sutured to the septal angle.

The graft is molded to the desired contour by finger manipulations using both hands. Then, a paper tape and a thermoplastic splint are used for fixation, while the splint is maintained for 1 week. If reshaping of the graft should require, after removing the splint on the seventh day, the split would be kept for a longer period. **Fig. 22** shows an example case of dorsal augmentation using the diced cartilage wrapped in temporal fascia.

Complications of Diced Cartilage Graft

Diced cartilage grafts allow for a relatively easy dorsal augmentation, which even the inexperienced operator can perform. Nevertheless, predictable adverse reactions include graft deviation, irregularity or focal depression, possible resorption, and visibility of the particle graft through the thin skin (cobble stone appearance).[23] In particular, focal depression (step-off) of the supratip may occur owing to technical difficulties in meticulous handling of the contact area between the dorsal graft and tip cartilage. If feasible, leaving the graft longer is desired to prevent this

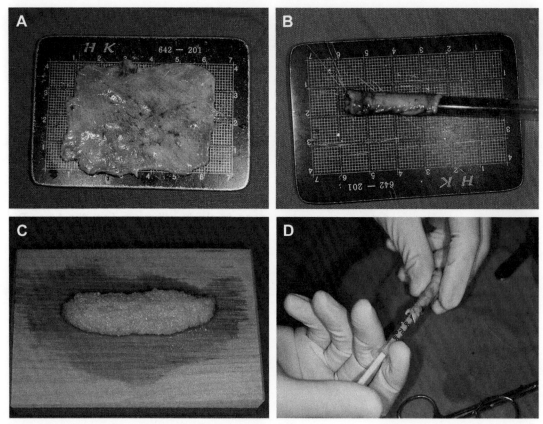

Fig. 21. Procedure of diced cartilage wrapped in temporal fascia. (*A*) Harvested deep temporal fascia. (*B*) A 1-mL syringe without a hub is wrapped with the temporal fascia. (*C*) Diced costal cartilage. (*D*) The diced cartilage particles in the syringe is slowly and gently infused and packed into the fascia tube.

problem; it is important to harvest a sufficiently long temporal fascia to do so. If the step-off is seen or palpated, the operator should place additional diced cartilage or a fascia graft.[16] Visibility of cartilage particles is rare among Asians with thick skin. However, a large cartilage particle graft on the thin skinned nose may be seen through the skin or show irregularities. For a thin-skinned nose, the cartilage must be diced in a much smaller size and the graft needs another layer of the fascia to wrap.[16] Minor irregularities may be corrected by morselizing the cartilage particles with a No. 16 needle via percutaneous puncture.[16] Daniel and associates[16,20] reported that overcorrection should not be necessary because the graft would not be absorbed, but the issue of resorption is controversial with numerous opinions from various authors.[24–26] The resorption rate of the diced cartilage graft is much less than that of ether the fascia graft or dermofat graft. However, partial resorption must be considered. Minimizing the

dead space among the particles by finely dicing the cartilage and maximally packing the particles into the temporal fascia tube would curtail dorsal height reduction as time passes.[24]

Advantages and Indications of Diced Cartilage Graft

Diced cartilage has many advantages.[16] Above all else, the operation is not technically demanding and opens up the use of this graft even to the inexperienced surgeons.

Compared with the block costal cartilage graft, the diced cartilage graft is much easier to fit the dorsal irregularity. Compared with the costal cartilage block graft, the diced cartilage graft has less tendency of the graft contour visibility through the skin, and no graft warping.

Molding to correct deviation, irregularities, or the width of a graft is possible for up to 2 weeks after surgery.

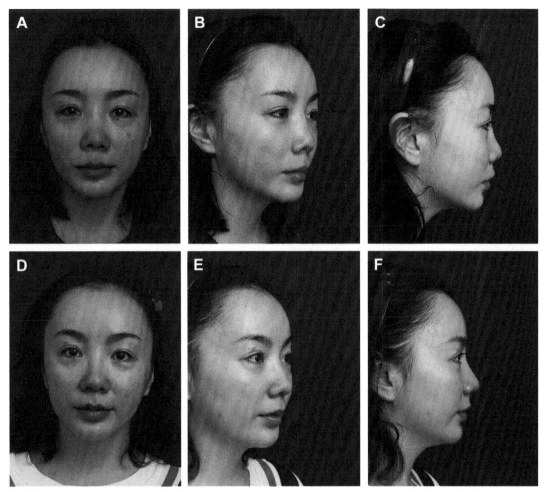

Fig. 22. Dorsal augmentation using diced cartilage wrapped up in the temporal fascia. (*A–C*) This female patient has a flat dorsum, especially on the mid-vault. (*D–F*) Eight months after surgery (dorsal augmentation surgery using the diced cartilage [costal cartilage]) wrapped in temporal fascia, and tip revisional surgery with the septal extension graft).

REFERENCES

1. Na DS, Jung SW, Kook KS, et al. Augmentation rhinoplasty with dermofat graft & fat injection. J Korean Soc Plast Reconstr Surg 2011;38(1):53–6.

2. Choi C, Kirk IS, Cho BC. Secondary augmentation rhinoplasty with immediate autogenous dermofat graft after removal of paraffinoma. J Korean Soc Plast Reconstr Surg 2007;034(06):785–91.

3. Hwang K, Kim DJ, Lee IJ. An anatomic comparison of the skin of five donor sites for dermal fat graft. Aesthetic Plast Surg 2001;46(3):327–31.

4. Little JW. Applications of the classic dermal fat graft in primary and secondary facial rejuvenation. Plast Reconstr Surg 2002;109(2):788–804.

5. Conley JJ, Clairmont AA. Dermal-fat-fascia grafts. Otolaryngology 1978;86(4 Pt 1). ORL-641-649.

6. Reich J. The application of dermis grafts in deformities of the nose. Plast Reconstr Surg 1983;71:772–82.

7. Erdogan B, Tuncel A, Adanali G, et al. Augmentation rhinoplasty with dermal graft and review of the literature. Plast Reconstr Surg 2003;111:2060–8.

8. Kim HK, Rhee SC. Augmentation rhinoplasty using a folded "pure" dermal graft. J Craniofac Surg 2013;24(5):1758–62.

9. Cho IC. Correction of contracted noses with unilateral cymbal cartilage and dermofat. 73rd congress of the Korean society of plastic and reconstructive surgeons, Seoul, Korea, November 14, 2015.

10. Jang YJ, Yu MS. Rhinoplasty for the Asian nose. Facial Plast Surg 2010;26(2):93–101.

11. Toriumi DM. Dorsal augmentation using autologous costal cartilage or microfat-infused soft tissue augmentation. Facial Plast Surg 2017;33(2):162–78.

12. Gunter JP, Clark CP, Friedman RM. Internal stabilization of autogenous rib cartilage grafts in rhinoplasty: a barrier to cartilage warping. Plast Reconstr Surg 1997;100:161–9.

13. Toriumi DM, Asher SA. Primary rhinoplasty techniques: use of costal cartilage. In: Cobo R, editor. Ethnic considerations in facial plastic surgery. Philadelphia: Thieme; 2016. p. 196–217.

14. Toriumi DM, Pero CD. Asian rhinoplasty. Clin Plast Surg 2010;37(2):335–52.

15. Toriumi DM. Discussion: use of autologous costal cartilage in Asian rhinoplasty. Plast Reconstr Surg 2012;130(6):1349–50.

16. Daniel RK. Diced cartilage grafts in rhinoplasty surgery: current techniques and applications. Plast Reconstr Surg 2008;122(6):1883–91.

17. Park JH, Jin HR. Use of autologous costal cartilage in Asian rhinoplasty. Plast Reconstr Surg 2012;130: 1338–48.

18. Balaji SM. Costal cartilage nasal augmentation rhinoplasty: study on warping. Ann Maxillofac Surg 2013;3:20–4.

19. Erol OO. The Turkish delight: a pliable graft for rhinoplasty. Plast Reconstr Surg 2000;105:2229–41.

20. Daniel RK, Calvert JW. Diced cartilage grafts in rhinoplastic surgery. Plast Reconstr Surg 2004;113: 2156–71.

21. Hoehne J, Gubisch W, Kreutzer C, et al. Refining the nasal dorsum with free diced cartilage. Facial Plast Surg 2016;32(4):345–50.

22. Kreutzer C, Hoehne J, Gubisch W, et al. Free diced cartilage: a new application of diced cartilage grafts in primary and secondary rhinoplasty. Plast Reconstr Surg 2017;140(3):461–70.

23. Park P, Jin HR. Diced cartilage in fascia for major nasal dorsal augmentation in Asians: a review of 15 consecutive cases. Aesthetic Plast Surg 2016;40:832–9.

24. Kelly MH, Bulstrode NW, Waterhouse N. Versatility of diced cartilage-fascia grafts in dorsal nasal augmentation. Plast Reconstr Surg 2007;120(6):1654–9.

25. Harel M, Margulis A. Dorsal augmentation with diced cartilage enclosed with temporal fascia in secondary endonasal rhinoplasty. Aesthet Surg J 2013; 33(6):809–16.

26. Fatemi MJ, Hasani ME, Rahimian S, et al. Survival of block and fascial-wrapped diced cartilage grafts: an experimental study in rabbits. Ann Plast Surg 2012; 69(3):326–30.

Homologous Tissue for Dorsal Augmentation

Chang-Hoon Kim, MD, PhD[a,b,]*, Sang Chul Park, MD[a]

KEYWORDS

- Asian rhinoplasty • Dorsal augmentation • Homologous grafts • Acellular dermal matrix
- Tutoplast-processed fascia lata

KEY POINTS

- Dorsal augmentation is the most commonly performed procedure in rhinoplasty for Asian patients.
- Homologous grafts derived from human tissues are safe and biocompatible.
- Acellular dermal matrix is a useful graft material owing to its long-term structural integrity and stability as well as low risk of infection or extrusion.
- Tutoplast-processed fascia lata is soft and easy to manipulate, providing a smooth postoperative contour of the nasal dorsum with low risk of infection or displacement.

INTRODUCTION

Dorsal augmentation is the most commonly performed procedure in rhinoplasty for Asian patients. Various materials are used for nasal dorsal augmentation, and surgeons continue to make efforts to find the ideal material. An ideal material is one that is safe and biocompatible with a low risk of complications, such as infection and displacement. Moreover, it should be easy to sculpt and mechanically stable with surrounding tissues.[1–4] Autologous grafts, including costal cartilage and conchal cartilage, have a high degree of biological tolerance; however, they have some drawbacks, such as donor site morbidity, long operation time, and potential difficulty in obtaining sufficient amounts for dorsal augmentation. Alloplastic implants, which are synthetic materials, including silicone, expanded polytetrafluoroethylene (Gore-Tex), and porous polyethylene (Medpor), have some shortcomings such as the risk of infection, contracture, and implant visibility. Therefore, homologous grafts derived from human tissues are recently receiving

the spotlight for their high degree of tissue tolerance and low infection risk. Furthermore, there is a limitation in selecting the augmentation materials when autologous grafts had been used in previous surgeries. In this situation, homologous grafts can be ideal graft materials. In this article, the authors describe the acellular dermal matrix (ADM) and Tutoplast-processed fascia lata (TPFL).

ACELLULAR DERMAL MATRIX
Characteristics of Acellular Dermal Matrix

ADM is a biocompatible, nonimmunogenic, off-the-shelf, and readily available material for dorsal augmentation.[5,6] ADM is processed from human cadaveric skin through specialized processing techniques. During its preparation, the epidermis and the cellular components of the dermis that can induce immune reactions are removed before freeze-drying.[1,7] The ADM is highly biocompatible because it preserves the essential structural components of the extracellular matrix, such as collagen and elastin fibers. Collagen and elastin, which are the main

Disclosure Statement: C-.H. Kim and S.C. Park have nothing to disclose.
[a] Department of Otorhinolaryngology, Yonsei University College of Medicine, 50 Yonsei-ro, Seodaemun-gu, Seoul 120-752, Korea; [b] The Airway Mucus Institute, Yonsei University College of Medicine, 50 Yonsei-ro, Seodaemun-gu, Seoul 120-752, Korea
* Corresponding author. Department of Otorhinolaryngology, Yonsei University College of Medicine, 50 Yonsei-ro, Seodaemun-gu, Seoul 120-752, Korea.
E-mail address: entman@yuhs.ac

Facial Plast Surg Clin N Am 26 (2018) 311–321
https://doi.org/10.1016/j.fsc.2018.03.005

components of ADM, provide tensile strength and elasticity. Maintaining the 3-dimensional natural dermal structures induce fibroblast infiltration and neovascularization, which promote tissue regeneration.[8,9] According to histologic analyses of implanted ADM, collagen and elastin fibers become denser, the expression of extracellular matrix proteins increases, and microvessel formation within ADM increases, whereas the thickness of the implanted ADM does not decrease over time.[7,10] These characteristics allow adequate tissue ingrowth and provide long-term structural integrity, which make displacement and exposure rare.

The most commonly used matrices are AlloDerm (LifeCell Corp, Branchburg, NJ, USA) and Mega-Derm (L&C BIO, Seongnam-si, Gyeonggi-do, Korea). The main differences of MegaDerm are its cross-linked structure and electron beam (e-beam) irradiation. The cross-linking of the collagen structure is important for long-term durability and strength. It enables reducing resorption and improving fibroblast infiltration into the dermal matrix, which allow MegaDerm to retain its rigidity and shape.[7,8,11,12] Gamma irradiation is used as a sterilization process for AlloDerm, whereas e-beam irradiation is done for MegaDerm. E-beam irradiation, which is a form of ionizing irradiation similar to gamma irradiation, creates more stable dermis tissue cross-link. E-beam irradiation (25 kGy) results in increased tension and elasticity.[7,13]

Types of Acellular Dermal Matrix

Various types of ADM have been introduced since its development in the early 1990s.[14,15] ADM has been used as a soft tissue replacement in reconstructive surgery, such as breast reconstruction, abdominal wall repair, burn management, and in combination with autologous thin split-thickness skin graft. In rhinoplasty, it is used in the nasal dorsum and the tip. For the nasal dorsum, it is useful for dorsal augmentation,[5,6,16,17] correction of dorsal irregularity,[18] and wrapping of autologous grafts or alloplastic implants for decreasing implant visibility, especially in patients with thin skin.[19–21]

There are 3 types of ADM according to characteristics. The carving type (the type generally used in dorsal augmentation) has a boat shape based on the shape of the nasal dorsum. It is 1 × 5 cm

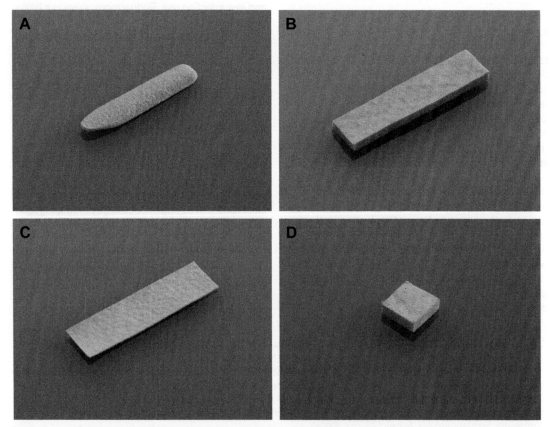

Fig. 1. Types of MegaDerm. (*A*) The carving type and (*B*) the block type are used for dorsal augmentation. (*C*) The block type is used for tip surgery. (*D*) The sheet type is used for wrapping of autologous grafts or alloplastic implants. (*Courtesy of* L&C Bio, Gyeonggi-do, South Korea; with permission.)

in size and has thicknesses of 3, 4, and 5 mm (**Fig. 1A**). The block type is cut by the surgeon according to the desired size and is used for dorsum (**Fig. 1B**) or tip augmentation (**Fig. 1C**). The sheet type is used as a wrapping material for the autologous grafts or alloplastic implants (**Fig. 1D**).

Surgical Procedure

ADM can be placed through the open approach or the endonasal approach. Before dorsal augmentation, it is helpful to mark the midline of the nasal dorsum and the new rhinion where the ADM would be placed. The skin flap over the nasal dorsum is elevated via careful dissection, keeping the dissection superficial to the perichondrium of the upper and lower lateral cartilage. The periosteum overlying the nasal bone is included in the skin flap by developing a subperiosteal plane at the junction of the upper lateral cartilage and nasal bone. It is important to keep this subperiosteal plane to prevent the displacement and visibility of the ADM after operation. Dissection is continued to the nasion in bilateral symmetry from the midline of the nasal dorsum. The pocket of the inserted ADM is created

a little larger than the size of ADM. When selecting the type of ADM product, the anticipated length and thickness of the ADM for appropriate augmentation according to the patient's dorsal height should be considered before surgery. The ADM should be held gently with bayonet forceps while placing the triangular portion toward the cephalic part. The suitability of the length and thickness of the ADM over the nasal dorsum should also be checked (**Fig. 2A**). When modification is needed, additional trimming can be easily done with the 15th blade. The ADM is inserted into the pocket in the nasal dorsum and gently placed into a suitable position under direct vision (**Fig. 2B**). After covering the skin flap, the height and shape of the nasal dorsum are confirmed once more, followed by skin closure (**Fig. 2C**). In most cases, ADM fixation with sutures is not necessary. However, the ADM can be sutured to surrounding structures, such as the upper lateral cartilage, as needed. The ADM may also be fixed with the skin from outside of the nose, maintaining the fixation for 1 week.

Although the ADM is used alone in dorsal augmentation, it can also be used with other alloplastic implants because of its low rigidity and

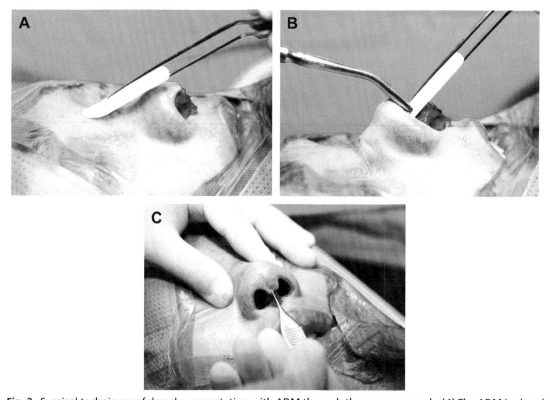

Fig. 2. Surgical techniques of dorsal augmentation with ADM through the open approach. (*A*) The ADM is placed above the nasal dorsum to check the suitability of its length and thickness for the nasal dorsum. (*B*) The ADM is inserted into the nasal dorsum and gently placed into a suitable position. (*C*) After covering the skin flap, the height and shape of the nasal dorsum are checked once more, followed by skin closure.

potential for absorption. For example, ADM and with alloplastic implant can be used in patients who need large amounts of thickness owing to severe saddle nose. As the ADM can be easily engaged with the surrounding tissues, it can help in fixing the inserted silicone or expanded polytetrafluoroethylene into the dorsum without displacement.

Advantage

ADM is an off-the-shelf product that is readily available and affordable.[5,16] Because the carving type designed for the shape of the nose has various thicknesses, the thickness desired for augmentation can be easily adjusted. The sheet type is easy to design into a suitable shape according to the surgical need. As the ADM has good elasticity and extensibility, trimming or manipulation can be done during the operation. It can provide a natural appearance to the skin, even in thin-skinned patients, owing to its softness and low rigidity. Because the ADM has a color similar to the skin and is not shiny, it can be used on top of other autologous grafts or alloplastic implants to compensate for the disadvantages of other implants.[1,5,16–18] Among patients who received revision rhinoplasty, the previously inserted implants may be palpable or visible and

dorsal nasal irregularity may occur. The ADM can be effectively used to correct various types of dorsal nasal irregularity because it has various thicknesses and a high resilience.

The greatest advantage of ADM is that it is a biocompatible material derived from human skin. It maintains the structure and the integrity of dermis, supporting tissue incorporation and rapid revascularization after implantation. These merits allow a natural appearance of the nose and adequate tissue ingrowth without graft migration. It is also safe and carries low risk of infection or foreign body reaction owing to the specialized manufacturing process removing cell debris, antigens, and potential viruses.[5–8,10]

Sherris and Oriel[6] reported the safety and efficacy of AlloDerm in 51 patients. In their study, there were no cases of infection, seroma formation, significant resorption, or extrusion. Gryskiewicz[5] reported that AlloDerm is natural and incorporated into surrounding tissue without infection or foreign body reaction.[16]

The presenting authors have used MegaDerm in dorsal augmentation for 120 patients. Postoperatively, most of the patients showed favorable results of dorsal augmentation on external nasal physical examination and endoscopic finding (**Figs. 3–5**). No serious complications, such as

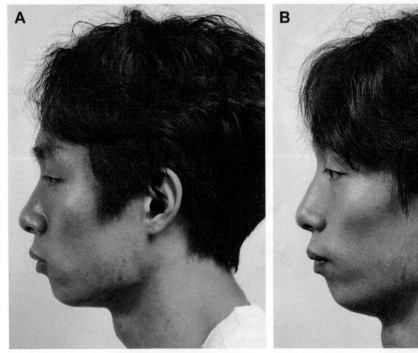

Fig. 3. Facial photographs of a 24-year-old male patient who underwent dorsal augmentation using MegaDerm. Dorsal augmentation and medial and lateral osteotomies were done through the endonasal approach. (*A*) Preoperative lateral view. (*B*) Postoperative lateral view taken 6 months postoperatively. Proper dorsal augmentation was accomplished after surgery.

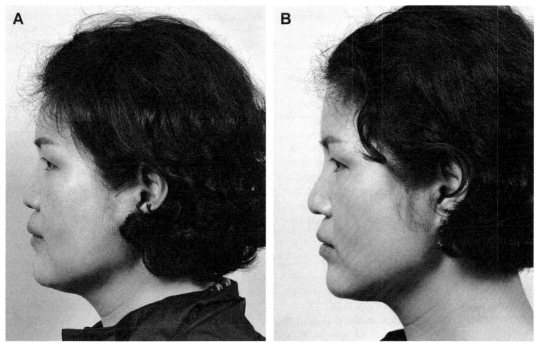

Fig. 4. Facial photographs of a 46-year-old female patient who underwent revision rhinoplasty with dorsal augmentation using MegaDerm. The silicone that had been placed 10 years ago was extruded in the right vestibule. The silicone was removed and replaced with MegaDerm. Medial and lateral osteotomies and tip plasty with septal extension graft were done through the open approach. (A) Preoperative lateral view. (B) Postoperative lateral view taken 6 months postoperatively. Proper dorsal augmentation was accomplished after surgery.

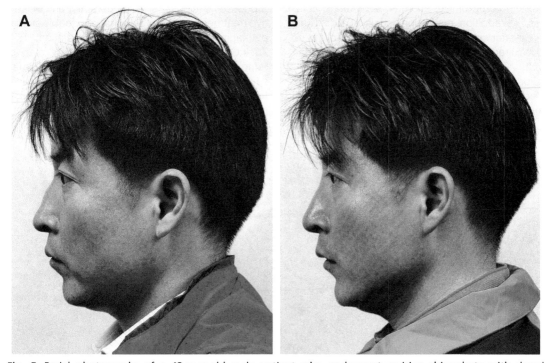

Fig. 5. Facial photographs of a 43-year-old male patient who underwent revision rhinoplasty with dorsal augmentation using MegaDerm. Hump removal, and medial and lateral osteotomies were done through the endonasal approach. (A) Preoperative lateral view. (B) Postoperative lateral view taken 6 months postoperatively. Proper dorsal augmentation was accomplished after surgery.

infection, foreign body reaction, or graft extrusion, were observed.

Moreover, the postoperative histologic changes of the implanted MegaDerm were examined in 4 patients who removed MegaDerm for proper aesthetic correction, not for graft-related complication. In all cases, the grafts were softly incorporated into the surrounding tissue without signs of infection. The stiffness and thickness of the graft did not change remarkably. On microscopic examination, the main portion consisted of collagen and elastin fibers, and newly formed vascular structure was detected in the periphery of the collagen tissues. There was no evidence of foreign body reaction, giant cells, and thick capsule formation (**Fig. 6**).

Disadvantage and Consideration

The resorption of the graft is considered the main problem of AlloDerm. Although there was no complete resorption, partial resorption of the graft has been proven. Forty-five percent of the patients showed partial graft resorption within the first 12 months.[17] In a study of 25 patients with revision rhinoplasty, 20% to 30% resorption over the bony dorsum and 10% to 15% over the tip were reported.[16] Resorption is more common in thin-skinned patients and those with preexisting vascular compromise, such as nasal telangiectasias.[10] In addition, resorption usually occurs within 1 year after surgery; thus, at least 1-year follow-up is required to evaluate the safety of implanted graft.[5]

For MegaDerm, there is one case report of infected nasal tip in a patient who underwent dorsum and tip augmentation with MegaDerm.[22]

According to the authors' experiences of Mega-Derm, graft displacement occurred in 2.5% of the patients. Moreover, partial resorption was observed in 2.5% of the patients.

TUTOPLAST-PROCESSED FASCIA LATA
Characteristics of Tutoplast-Processed Fascia Lata

Autologous fascia grafts, including the temporalis fascia and the fascia lata, have been used in rhinoplasty for dorsal augmentation and onlay camouflage graft.[23,24] Compared with the temporalis fascia, the fascia lata can provide an abundant amount of tissue with significant thickness for dorsal augmentation. However, harvesting autologous fascia lata needs an additional incision and procedure. The autologous fascia lata decreases in volume as it dries, and it can be difficult to manipulate in wet condition. Therefore, homologous fascia, such as TPFL, was introduced with the advantage of avoiding the donor site morbidity and reducing operation time.[25,26]

The representative products of TPFL are Tutoplast fascia lata (Tutoplast; Tutogen Medical GmbH, Neunkirchen am Brand, Germany) and Allosheet (CG Bio, Seongnam-si, Gyeonggi-do, Korea). They undergo Tutoplast tissue sterilization processes, including alkaline, osmotic, and oxidative treatments, solvent dehydration, double sterile packaging, and finally, gamma irradiation (15–25 kGy). These validated processing stages remove immunogenic structures and pathogens, while preserving biochemical integrity and native tissue structures.[26,27] Bioimplants by the Tutoplast process have been applied in orthopedic,

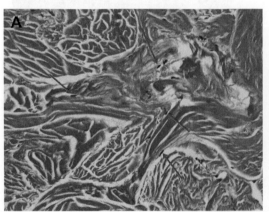
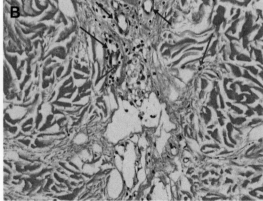

Fig. 6. Histologic examination of the implanted MegaDerm at 1 year postoperatively. Hematoxylin-eosin staining at ×200. (*A*) The structure was mainly composed of dense collagen tissue, with infiltration of a few fibroblasts (*green arrows*). (*B*) Newly formed vessels (*blue arrows*) were identified in the periphery of the collagen tissues. There were a few infiltrating lymphocytes (*red arrows*).

abdominal, plastic, ophthalmologic, and urologic surgery.[28] In rhinoplasty, TPFL has been used in dorsal augmentation, tip surgery, and reconstruction of the paranasal sinuses and nasal dorsum.[29–33] The use of TPFL in dorsal augmentation is safe and effective, especially providing a smooth postoperative contour of the nasal dorsum with low risk of infection.

Surgical Procedure

Starting with skin incision, supraperichondrial dissection of the cartilaginous dorsum and subperiosteal dissection of the bony dorsum are clearly made. The upper end of the material should be placed at the midcorneal level, and the lower end placed at the supratip area under the lower lateral crura. TPFL is rehydrated in saline solution for at least 5 minutes before use (according to the manufacturer's instructions) and then cut into multiple long strips 1 cm in width. The strips are usually layered (2 to 7 layers in the literature[29,33–35]) and sutured together with 5-0 polydioxanone, according to the required dorsal augmentation (**Fig. 7**). It is better for the

cephalic end of TPFL having a stepladder contour for smooth elevation of the radix. Careful beveling is needed to avoid the graft visibility in the radix area. The stack of layered TPFL are rounded off and inserted into the nasal dorsum. When further augmentation of nasal dorsum is required, crushed septal cartilage or diced conchal cartilage may be placed under TPFL.[34] In addition, septal cartilage or bone might be sandwiched between layers of TPFL and held together with separate absorbable sutures for ease of the graft insertion and the subsequent manipulation in endonasal approach of dorsal augmentation.[36]

Advantage

TPFL is easy to manipulate, such as cutting into the desired shape and making multilayer stacks. It is available in a variety of sizes and can be designed depending on the desired shape of nasal dorsum. Furthermore, it is a biocompatible and safe graft with low risk of displacement or extrusion. Delayed infection is very rare compared with the alloplastic implants. Once TPFL is

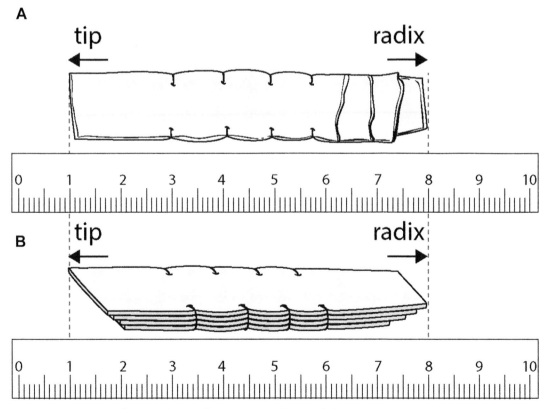

Fig. 7. The illustration of 4-layered TPFL after suturing with 5-0 polydioxanone. (*A*) Basal view and (*B*) lateral view of TPFL. (*Courtesy of* Dong-Su Jang, Seoul, Medical Illustrator, South Korea.)

engrafted, there is little chance of infection. More-over, its soft contour enables conforming well to the surrounding tissue, resulting in smooth contour of nasal dorsum.

In a study of 69 patients who underwent dorsal augmentation with TPFL alone or in combination with other materials, no serious complications, such as infection, graft extrusion, or graft visibility, were observed during mean follow-up of 17 months.[29] In the research of revision rhino-plasty with TPFL, 88% of the patients showed favorable aesthetic improvement without major complications.[35]

The presenting authors experienced 104 pa-tients treated with dorsal augmentation with TPFL. Proper augmentation of the dorsal and radix area was attained in both primary and revision rhi-noplasty (**Figs. 8** and **9**). There were no cases of infection, graft displacement, or significant resorption.[33]

Furthermore, the postoperative histologic changes of the implanted TPFL were investigated in 2 patients who removed TPFL for proper aesthetic correction, not for graft-related compli-cations. In both cases, the grafts were softly incor-porated into the surrounding tissue without signs of infection or seroma. The thickness of TPFL did not decrease significantly, maintaining favorable shape. On microscopic examination, the structure was mainly composed of dense fibrous tissue with neovascularization and fibroblast proliferation. The graft conformed well to the surrounding tissue accompanied by fibrosis at the peripheral area. There was no evidence of thick capsule formation (**Fig. 10**).

Disadvantage and Consideration

The major disadvantage of TPFL is resorption over time. In a study of a rabbit rhinoplasty model, there was no significant thickness reduction in both TPFL and autologous fascia lata grafts for 6 months.[37] However, surgeons should keep in mind the possibility of resorption when using TPFL in humans. The resorption rate is different in each patient, 0.7% and 4.3% reported in the studies of Jang and colleagues.[29,34] According to the report by Altun and colleagues,[35] major and minimal resorption rates were 7.1% and 21.4%, respectively, in the patients with revision rhinoplasty. Mechanisms of TPFL absorption include host-versus-graft reaction, inward growth of surrounding connective tissue, and volume reduction by surrounding tissue pressure.

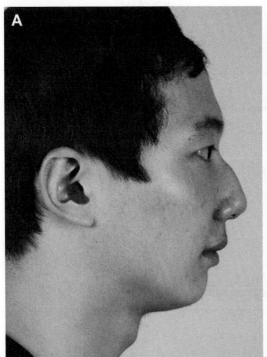
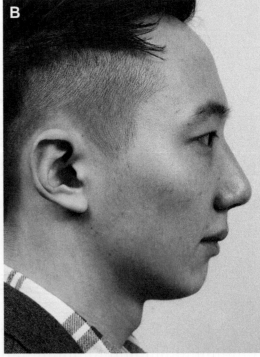

Fig. 8. Facial photographs of a male patient who underwent dorsal augmentation using TPFL. (*A*) Preoperative lateral view. (*B*) Postoperative lateral view taken 6 months postoperatively. Proper dorsal augmentation was accomplished after surgery.

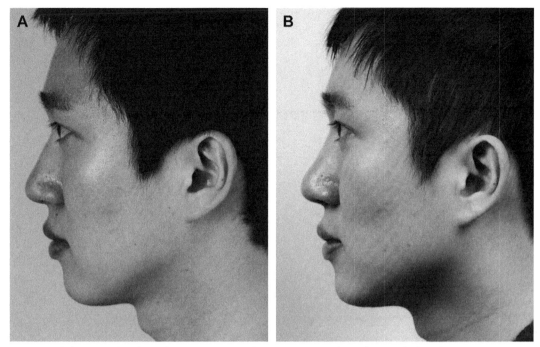

Fig. 9. Facial photographs of a male patient who underwent revision rhinoplasty with dorsal augmentation using TPFL. (*A*) Preoperative lateral view. (*B*) Postoperative lateral view taken 6 months postoperatively. Proper dorsal augmentation was accomplished after surgery.

Infection is a rare complication. One case has been reported by Kang and colleagues,[38] but it seems to be due to contamination of bacteria during surgery rather than the problem of TPFL itself.

The presenting authors experienced 5 cases (4.8%) of dorsal irregularity at 6 months postoperatively; however, this phenomenon was resolved without any surgical intervention in 4 cases (**Fig. 11**). Considering the short time taken for spontaneous resolution, the irregularity may be due to simple crumpling during the natural healing process of the nasal dorsum area. In addition, there were 4 cases (3.8%) of skin telangiectasia; all of them have recovered after laser therapy.

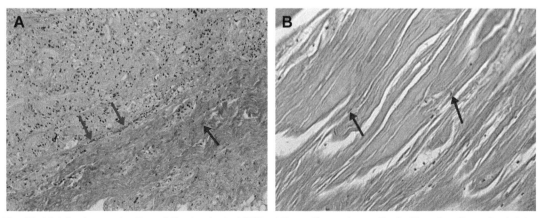

Fig. 10. Histologic examination of the implanted TPFL at 7 months postoperatively. Hematoxylin-eosin staining at ×100 (*A*) and ×200 (*B*) showed dense fibrous tissue with neovascularization (*red arrows*) and fibroblast infiltration (*blue arrows*).

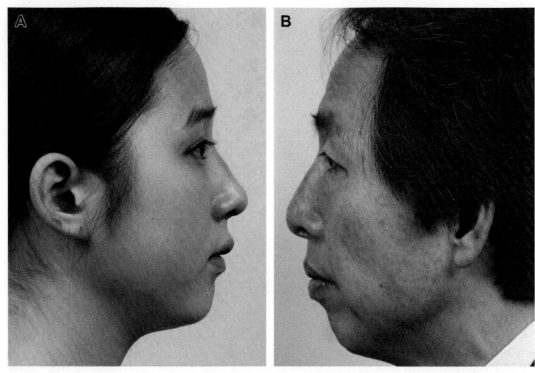

Fig. 11. The irregularity of nasal dorsum after primary (*A*) and revision (*B*) augmentation rhinoplasty using TPFL.

SUMMARY

Dorsal augmentation is an essential procedure in rhinoplasty especially for Asian patients; thus, it is important to find the ideal augmentation material. Homologous graft materials are safe and biocompatible with a low risk of complications, such as infection and extrusion. ADM is processed from human skin through specialized processing techniques, preserving the structure and the integrity of dermis. ADM provides a natural appearance of the nose and long-term structural integrity without extrusion. Most of the patients with ADM showed favorable results without serious complications. TPFL is derived from fascia lata that underwent sterilization processes. TPFL is soft and easy to manipulate, providing a smooth postoperative contour of the nasal dorsum with low risk of infection or displacement. It conforms well to the surrounding tissue, accompanied by satisfactory aesthetic results without major complications. Resorption of the graft is considered the main problem in both ADM and TPFL. Care should be taken especially in thin-skinned patients and those with preexisting vascular compromise. Taken together, homologous grafts, ADM and TPFL, are feasible graft materials that deliver adequate augmentation and patient satisfaction with minimal complications in both primary and revision rhinoplasty.

REFERENCES

1. Romo T 3rd, Kwak ES. Nasal grafts and implants in revision rhinoplasty. Facial Plast Surg Clin North Am 2006;14(4):373–87, vii.
2. Jang YJ, Moon BJ. State of the art in augmentation rhinoplasty: implant or graft? Curr Opin Otolaryngol Head Neck Surg 2012;20(4):280–6.
3. Brenner MJ, Hilger PA. Grafting in rhinoplasty. Facial Plast Surg Clin North Am 2009;17(1):91–113, vii.
4. Malone M, Pearlman S. Dorsal augmentation in rhinoplasty: a survey and review. Facial Plast Surg 2015;31(3):289–94.
5. Gryskiewicz JM. Dorsal augmentation with AlloDerm. Semin Plast Surg 2008;22(2):90–103.
6. Sherris DA, Oriel BS. Human acellular dermal matrix grafts for rhinoplasty. Aesthet Surg J 2011; 31(7 Suppl):95S–100S.
7. Lee JH, Kim HG, Lee WJ. Characterization and tissue incorporation of cross-linked human acellular dermal matrix. Biomaterials 2015;44:195–205.
8. Carlson TL, Lee KW, Pierce LM. Effect of cross-linked and non-cross-linked acellular dermal matrices on the expression of mediators involved in wound healing and matrix remodeling. Plast Reconstr Surg 2013;131(4):697–705.
9. Cummings LC, Kaldahl WB, Allen EP. Histologic evaluation of autogenous connective tissue and acellular dermal matrix grafts in humans. J Periodontol 2005;76(2):178–86.

10. Sajjadian A, Naghshineh N, Rubinstein R. Current status of grafts and implants in rhinoplasty: part II. homologous grafts and allogenic implants. Plast Reconstr Surg 2010;125(3):99e–109e.

11. Dunn RM. Cross-linking in biomaterials: a primer for clinicians. Plast Reconstr Surg 2012;130(5 Suppl 2): 18S–26S.

12. Cole PD, Stal D, Sharabi SE, et al. A comparative, long-term assessment of four soft tissue substitutes. Aesthet Surg J 2011;31(6):674–81.

13. Seto A, Gatt CJ Jr, Dunn MG. Radioprotection of tendon tissue via crosslinking and free radical scavenging. Clin Orthop Relat Res 2008;466(8):1788–95.

14. Megaderm. L&C Bio. Product. Available at: http://lncbio.co.kr/product/megaderm/. Accessed September 1, 2017.

15. AlloDerm. Lifecell Corp. Product. Available at: http://www.lifecell.com/products/allodermtm. Accessed September 1, 2017.

16. Gryskiewicz JM. Waste not, want not: the use of AlloDerm in secondary rhinoplasty. Plast Reconstr Surg 2005;116(7):1999–2004.

17. Gryskiewicz JM, Rohrich RJ, Reagan BJ, et al. The use of AlloDerm for the correction of nasal contour deformities. Plast Reconstr Surg 2001; 107(2):561–70.

18. Jackson I, Yavuzer R. AlloDerm for dorsal nasal irregularities. Plast Reconstr Surg 2001;107(2):553–8.

19. Suh MK, Lee KH, Harijan A, et al. Augmentation rhinoplasty with silicone implant covered with acellular dermal matrix. J Craniofac Surg 2017;28(2):445–8.

20. Gordon CR, Alghoul M, Goldberg JS, et al. Diced cartilage grafts wrapped in AlloDerm for dorsal nasal augmentation. J Craniofac Surg 2011;22(4): 1196–9.

21. Romo T, Sclafani AP, Sabini P. Reconstruction of the major saddle nose deformity using composite alloimplants. Facial Plast Surg 1998;14(02):151–7.

22. Lee KH. Infection in the nasal tip caused by acellular dermal matrix. Plast Reconstr Surg Glob Open 2015; 3(12):e581.

23. Karaaltin MV, Orhan KS, Demirel T. Fascia lata graft for nasal dorsal contouring in rhinoplasty. J Plast Reconstr Aesthet Surg 2009;62(10):1255–60.

24. Baker TM, Courtiss EH. Temporalis fascia grafts in open secondary rhinoplasty. Plast Reconstr Surg 1994;93(4):802–10.

25. Sclafani AP, McCormick SA, Cocker R. Biophysical and microscopic analysis of homologous dermal and fascial materials for facial aesthetic and reconstructive uses. Arch Facial Plast Surg 2002; 4(3):164–71.

26. Gubisch W, Constantinescu MA. Refinements in extracorporal septoplasty. Plast Reconstr Surg 1999; 104(4):1131–9 [discussion: 1140].

27. lata Tpf. Tutogen Medical GmbH. Product. Available at: http://www.rtix.com/en_us/healthcare-professionals/tissue-sterilization/tutoplast-tissue-sterilization-process. Accessed September 1, 2017.

28. Ghoniem GM. Allograft sling material: is it the state of the art? Int Urogynecol J 2000;11(2):69–70.

29. Jang YJ, Wang JH, Sinha V, et al. Tutoplast-processed fascia lata for dorsal augmentation in rhinoplasty. Otolaryngol Head Neck Surg 2007;137(1): 88–92.

30. Kim JH, Wang JH, Jang YJ. Excision of a nasal dermoid sinus cyst via open rhinoplasty approach and primary reconstruction using tutoplast-processed fascia lata. Clin Exp Otorhinolaryngol 2010;3(1): 48–51.

31. Jang YJ, Kim JH. Use of tutoplast-processed fascia lata as an onlay graft material for tip surgery in rhinoplasty. Otolaryngol Head Neck Surg 2011;144(4): 528–32.

32. Hyun SM, Min JY, Jang YJ. Reduction osteoplasty for treating pneumosinus dilatans of the maxillary sinus. J Laryngol Otol 2013;127(2):207–10.

33. Kim YS, Park DY, Shin DH, et al. Surgical outcomes of primary and revision augmentation rhinoplasty using a processed fascia lata. Am J Rhinol Allergy 2015;29(2):141–4.

34. Jang YJ, Song HM, Yoon YJ, et al. Combined use of crushed cartilage and processed fascia lata for dorsal augmentation in rhinoplasty for Asians. Laryngoscope 2009;119(6):1088–92.

35. Altun H, Hanci D, Can Y. Multilayer tutoplast-processed fascia lata use in revision rhinoplasty for overresected dorsum. Eur J Plast Surg 2015; 38(4):279–84.

36. Issing W, Anari S. Sandwich technique in nasal dorsal augmentation. Eur Arch Otorhinolaryngol 2011; 268(1):83–6.

37. Yu MS, Park HS, Lee HJ, et al. Histomorphological changes of Tutoplast-processed fascia lata grafts in a rabbit rhinoplasty model. Otolaryngol Head Neck Surg 2012;147(2):239–44.

38. Kang IG, Jung JH, Cha HE, et al. A case of infection of tutoplast-processed fascia lata in augmentation rhinoplasty. J Rhinol 2010;17(1):60–2.

Injection Rhinoplasty Using Filler

Hyoung Jin Moon, MD*

KEYWORDS

• Rhinoplasty • Filler • Injectables • Nose • Nonsurgical rhinoplasty • Injection rhinoplasty

KEY POINTS

- Filler must be injected into the deep fatty layer, between the perichondrium or periosteum and muscle layer, where important blood vessels are not located, to help avoid vascular compromise.
- Filler is usually injected in the order of the radix; rhinion; tip; and, finally, the supratip area.
- The surgeon should always mark the midline on the nasal bridge and perform the procedure without deviating from the midline to minimize asymmetry of the injected nasal dorsum.

INTRODUCTION

Rhinoplasty is among the most commonly performed operations in cosmetic surgery. It is performed more frequently among Asians owing to the low nasal bridge and flat tip. However surgical rhinoplasty using implants and autologous grafts require longer recovery time and have many complications; therefore, many patients hesitate to get the surgery.[1] Also, it is well-recognized that there is a steep learning curve for rhinoplasty. For these reasons, many doctors and patients prefer a simpler and cheaper procedure with fewer side effects and a shorter down time. Rhinoplasty using filler is the procedure that meets this demand.[2]

Fillers by definition, refers to all substances that can increase volume by injection. The most well-known types of fillers include hyaluronic acid products, collagen, paraffin, and liquid silicon. Fillers are usually classified by their components.

Fillers also can be classified by duration of their effects. Fillers with a duration of less than 2 years are called temporary fillers, those with a duration of 2 to 5 years are called semipermanent fillers, and those lasting no less than 5 years after injection are called permanent fillers.

Most of the fillers have a good safety profile. However, serious side effects, such as granuloma formation or inflammation, have been reported with several filler products; therefore, it is necessary to select the ideal filler by understanding the characteristics of each product. The ideal filler should have no tissue reaction; be long-lasting, safe, and easy to inject; and have no intratissue migration or allergic reaction.

ANATOMY FOR INJECTION RHINOPLASTY USING FILLER

Injection rhinoplasty using filler can only be successfully performed if the nasal anatomy is thoroughly understood. It is a procedure that sculpts the nasal shape by injecting materials in the space between the skin and nasal skeleton composed of cartilage and bone.

The solid frame of the nose is the supporting structure that maintains the shape of the injected filler and achieves an esthetic result. Therefore, a satisfactory result cannot be expected after the procedure if the frame of the nose is deformed or weakened. Rhinoplasty using filler can be said to reflect the personal ability of the surgeon, the anatomic characteristics of the patient's nose, and the surgeon's recognition of such individual variation. When performing rhinoplasty using filler, all aspects must be considered, including thickness and quality

Disclosure: The author has nothing to disclose.
Beup Aesthetic Plastic Surgery Clinic, Seoul, Republic of Korea
* 4F, Dongyang Building, 591, Sinsa-dong, Gangnam-gu, Seoul 06025, Republic of Korea.
E-mail address: Beautymoon@hotmail.co.kr

facialplastic.theclinics.com

of the skin and the soft tissue; and the size, shape and strength of the cartilage and bone.

Nasal Soft Tissue

It is important to assess the nasal skin before performing filler rhinoplasty. In general, Asian patients have thicker, oilier skin and more subcutaneous tissue than white patients.

It may be more difficult to perform filler rhinoplasty on patients with thick, oily skin because they may experience severe postprocedure edema more often and because creating a pleasing 3-dimensional shape is challenging. On the other hand, in such patients, minute irregularities or asymmetry can be camouflaged more easily compared with patients with thin skin.

The soft tissue of the nasal bridge is the thickest at the nasion, and the thinnest is at the rhinion, which is the junction of the upper lateral cartilages and the nasal bones.[3]

The part of external nose between the skin and bone or cartilages consists of 4 layers: the superficial fatty layer, the fibromuscular layer (SMAS [superficial musculo-aponeurotic system] layer), the deep fatty layer, and the perichondrium or perichondrium.[4]

Major blood vessels of the external nose are in the SMAS layer or the superficial fatty layer.[5] Therefore, to minimize vascular injuries, the ideal and safe layer for filler injection is the deep fatty layer located between the SMAS and the perichondrium or periosteum (**Fig. 1**).

Sometimes some of nasal muscles are paralyzed using botulinum toxin to enhance the effect of rhinoplasty using filler. For example, the depressor septi nasi muscle originates from the orbicularis oris and terminates at the medial crura of the lower lateral cartilage. This muscle lowers the nasal tip when smiling or making a facial expression, and it is often paralyzed by injecting botulinum toxin to inhibit the function.[6]

Vascular Supply of the External Nose

The most feared complication of filler injection is intraarterial embolization into the blood vessel. To prevent this complication, the surgeon must be familiar with the blood supply of the nose.

Both the internal carotid artery and the external carotid artery supply blood to the external nose via the ophthalmic artery and the facial artery, respectively. The ophthalmic artery mainly supplies blood to the upper part of the nose via the external nasal

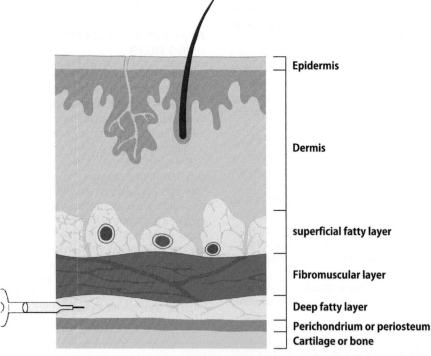

Epidermis

Dermis

superficial fatty layer

Fibromuscular layer

Deep fatty layer
Perichondrium or periosteum
Cartilage or bone

Fig. 1. The soft tissue of the nose consists of 4 layers: the superficial fatty layer, the fibromuscular layer (SMAS), the deep fatty layer, and the periosteum or perichondrium. Major blood vessels of the external nose are located in the superficial fatty layer (SMAS layer). Therefore, to minimize vascular injuries, the ideal and safe layer for filler injection is the deep fatty layer located between the SMAS and the perichondrium or periosteum. (*From* Moon HJ. Use of fillers in rhinoplasty. Clin Plast Surg 2016;43(1):307–17; with permission.)

branch of the anterior ethmoid artery and the dorsal nasal artery; the facial artery gives rise to the angular and superior labial arteries that supply the lower part of the nose. Each of these branches out to the lateral nasal artery and the columellar artery. The nasal tip receives blood supply from the dorsal nasal artery superiorly and the lateral nasal artery and the columellar artery inferiorly.

SELECTION OF PATIENTS

To carry out injection rhinoplasty using filler effectively, the surgeon must select patients who are suitable for rhinoplasty using filler. The patients who generally tend to show good results are those with mild hump nose, mildly deviated nose, high nasal tip with flat radix, slight imbalance from surgery, and so forth. Those with a severe hump nose, severely deviated nose, upturned nose, and bulbous nose are not expected to have good results from filler alone.

One should be cautious when offering this procedure to patients who have had nasal implants inserted, or those with history of paraffin or liquid silicon injections, because skin irregularities and vascular compromise may occur.

INJECTION TECHNIQUE

Rhinoplasty using filler comprises 2 main parts: injecting over the nasal dorsum and injection the tip. Relatively solid and firm structures support the nasal dorsum, namely, the nasal bones and the upper lateral cartilages, so it is easier to augment with filler injection. However, it is not easy to project or lengthen the nasal tip, especially in Asian patients owing to weak supporting structures.

After comparing and analyzing the ideal nose shape and the patient's nose shape, decide which part is to be raised and by how much.

Applying local anesthetic ointment for about 40 minutes is usually sufficient for anesthesia before the procedure.

The midline is marked along the nasal dorsum after anesthesia. It should be marked accurately to prevent complications such as asymmetry. To find the starting point that forms the ideal nasofrontal angle is very important. The nasal radix should begin at the level of supratarsal fold on lateral view in Asian patients but it varies depending on the preference of the patient, height of the forehead, and the length of the nose.[7] The nasal dorsum should lie 1 to 2 mm below a line drawn from the nasion to the nasal tip for both the Asian and white patients.[8] However, some patients may prefer a straight nasal bridge.

The nose can be divided into 4 parts for the procedure: radix, rhinion, supratip, and tip (**Fig. 2**). Different injection methods should be used because each part has a different thickness of the subcutaneous tissue, as well as different characteristics and strength of supporting structures. After marking the 4 sections, any defect that requires filler injection on either side of the nose should be marked out.

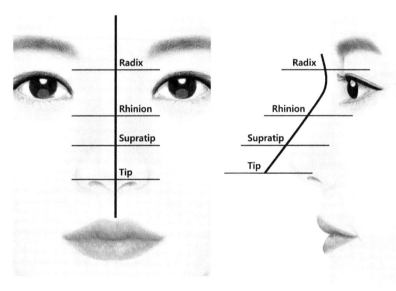

Fig. 2. The surgeon marks the nasal midline on the nasal dorsum before the procedure. The midline line must be marked accurately to prevent complications such as asymmetry. The next step is to mark the point of the ideal radix position. In Asian patients, this is the supratarsal crease. The filler procedure is performed by dividing the nose into 4 sections: radix, rhinion, supratip, and tip. Different injection methods must be used because each part has different thickness of subcutaneous tissue, as well as different characteristics and strength of supporting structures. (*From* Moon HJ. Use of fillers in rhinoplasty. Clin Plast Surg 2016;43(1):307–17; with permission.)

Filler is usually injected in the order of the radix; the rhinion; the tip; and, finally, the supratip area (**Fig. 3**). The tip is injected before the supratip area because the tip supporting is weak, especially in Asian patients; thus it is difficult to predict the amount of projection that can be achieved. If the supratip area is injected before the nasal tip, and the surgeon is unable to achieve adequate tip projection thereafter, a Polly beak deformity may occur.

There are disadvantages for tip augmentation with filler injection, such as the short longevity or the limitation of projection that can be achieved compared with surgical rhinoplasty. However, this is a good alternative when the patient refuses surgery or wants a simple procedure that has minimal down time.[9]

The areas that are commonly injected when performing nasal tip contouring using filler are the nasal spine, the columellar space, the interdomal area, and the alar margin (**Fig. 4**).

Filling the area of the nasal spine has the effect of elevating the nasal tip by increasing the lifting capacity, which can alter an acute nasolabial angle to 1 that is more obtuse. Usually, approximately 0.5 ml of filler is used.[10]

If filler is injected into the columellar space, injected filler functions as a column to increase the support for the nasal tip, and can correct a retracted columella. Usually, 0.2 to 0.3 cm³ of filler is used. In the columella, the arterial vasculature is mostly located between the MC and the epidermis, so it will be better to inject filler between the medial crus (MC) to prevent vascular compromise.[11] When injecting filler into the nasal spine area, the membranous septum should be held with the fingers to keep the filler in the center and not let it budge from the membranous septum toward the nasal cavity. If the filler bulges from the membranous septum toward the nasal cavity, the patient may complain of nasal obstruction. Therefore, check whether the filler bulges into the nasal cavity after the procedure; if it does, move it to the center by molding.

Injecting the tip with filler creates volume for reshaping. The volume and location of injection depends on the desired appearance. Usually, about 0.2 cm³ is sufficient and injection into the subfibromuscular tissue is recommended. When injecting filler into the nasal tip, it is safer to inject in the midline to minimize tip deviation and asymmetry.

Alar retraction can be corrected through filler injection. However, it is not advised for patients who have scarring from previous surgery due to the risk of dermal necrosis or irregularities.

Injection filler rhinoplasty mostly uses the linear threading technique in which filler is injected as the needle or cannula is withdrawn after insertion. Surgeons can use a sharp needle or a blunt cannula; however, a blunt cannula is recommended for beginners because there is relatively less possibility of complications such as intravascular injection. Sometimes, a single injection is used to correct the local defect, using a .5 inch-long sharp needle.

The most important point in filler injection rhinoplasty is to perform the procedure properly so that the filler stays at the midline. The most common complaint after any rhinoplasty is asymmetry. This is also true of rhinoplasty using filler. As previously mentioned, the surgeon should always mark the midline on the nasal bridge and perform the procedure without deviating from the midline to minimize such complications.

It is strongly recommended that the surgeon use both hands when doing nose treatment with filler. While using 1 hand for injection, the noninjecting hand should guide the needle and product into the tissue. This ensures no spreading or diffusion of the product and, if necessary, the filler can be molded.[12]

After injection, it is recommended to form a smooth and dorsal contour by massaging and molding. Any area with excessive filler should be pressed toward the base and any area that is underfilled should have more filler injected. It is best to perform the touch-ups after 2 weeks because mild edema may occur after the procedure. No special dressings nor prescription for antibiotics are needed.

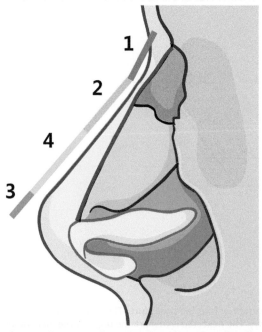

Fig. 3. Filler is usually injected in the order of radix, rhinion, tip, and supratip area. (*Adapted from* Moon HJ. Use of fillers in rhinoplasty. Clin Plast Surg 2016;43(1):307–17; with permission.)

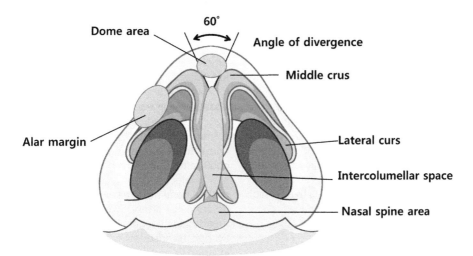

Fig. 4. The areas commonly injected when performing nasal tip augmentation using filler are the nasal spine, columellar space, interdomal area, and alar margin. The amount of filler injected to each part is about 0.2 to 0.5 cm³. (*Adapted from* Moon HJ. Use of fillers in rhinoplasty. Clin Plast Surg 2016;43(1):307–17; with permission.)

COMPLICATIONS

Injection rhinoplasty is very safe but, occasionally, complications may occur. Most complications can be prevented by selecting safe products and performing the procedure in an appropriate manner.

Major complications of filler injections are swelling, erythema, bruising, discoloration, irregularity, lumps, or granuloma formation. Infections may occur, and serious complications such as dermal necrosis due to vascular compromise are rare but possible as well.[13]

Bruising

Bruising is a common complication of filler injections; it is caused by vascular damage by a needle. To reduce bruising, piercing of muscular layers must be minimized during filler injection, the injection site should be cleaned with an alcohol swab, and the procedure should be performed in a bright room with adequate lighting. The patient should be informed not to take blood thinners such as aspirin 1 week before the procedure. Applying icepacks on the injection site immediately after helps to minimize bruising, and special needles or cannulae can be used to minimize vascular injury. If bleeding occurs during the procedure, the injection site is covered with gauze and pressed for several minutes to stop hematoma formation. The patient should be informed that bruising is only temporary and does not affect the final therapeutic effect. It should also be explained that the bruise can darken in the days following the injection but will slowly fade over about 10 days.

Asymmetry

Among the most common complications of rhinoplasty using filler is asymmetry. To prevent asymmetry, the needle tip must be placed precisely in the midline and the direction of the bevel should be toward the median plane. When injecting filler into a patient with a deviated nose, it is prudent to watch the shape of the nose closely while slowly injecting small amounts of filler.

Visible Implant

Injecting filler too superficially (close to the skin surface) may result in unevenness of the injected site or visibility of the filler. To avoid this, the filler should be injected into the appropriate layer according to its characteristics.[14]

Hypersensitivity

There may be hypersensitivity to the filler ingredients. The main symptoms are pain and erythema, accompanied by pruritus and fever. In most cases, the symptoms subside as the causative substance disappears. In severe cases, administering corticosteroid products and warm compression may help alleviate the symptoms. Many reactions that are assumed to be allergic or hypersensitivity responses are most likely caused by bacterial reactions.[15]

Granuloma or Nodule

Occasionally mass can form at the injected area after filler injection. These can be due to either granuloma or nodule formation. A granuloma is an immune response to an injected foreign body and is formed by accumulation of immune response-related cells, such as lymphocytes, to eliminate the foreign body. Treatment is with corticosteroid injection or surgical removal. Nodules are round and solid. Nodule development is a common complication following the use of fillers for soft tissue augmentation and is commonly categorized as inflammatory or noninflammatory in nature. Inflammatory nodules may appear anywhere from days to years after treatment, whereas noninflammatory nodules are typically seen immediately following injection and are usually secondary to improper placement of the filler.[16] Treatment is with hyaluronidase (if the filler used is hyaluronic acid), corticosteroid, or surgical removal.

Vascular Compromise

The most serious complications that occurs after rhinoplasty using filler are dermal necrosis and blindness. The mechanism leading to tissue necrosis after hyaluronic acid filler injection is not fully understood. Vascular compromise can be largely divided into intravascular or extravascular causes. Intravascular factors include direct obstruction of arteries by large-molecular-weight hyaluronic acid fillers and chemical damage of the endothelial lining by hyaluronic acid or impurities in the fillers.[17] Extravascular causes include external venous compression due to excessive volume of injection,[18] or edema and inflammatory response caused by a component of the filler.[19] Among the previously suggested factors, intraarterial obstruction is supported by many investigators as a main cause for vascular compromise after filler injection.

Intraarterial embolism

Cause Most cases of intraarterial embolism that occur after rhinoplasty using filler occur when the filler is injected directly into the dorsal nasal artery or the lateral nasal artery. This is especially of the dorsal nasal artery, which, as its name suggests, runs along the dorsum of the nose. The needle tip can be inserted into the blood vessel if it is inserted in parallel with the blood vessel. The dorsal nasal artery anastomoses with branches of facial artery so the widespread embolism through the connected blood vessels manifests as skin necrosis in a geographic pattern. It is also a branch of the ophthalmic artery, so propagation of the filler embolus may also cause eye symptoms. The lateral nasal artery is a branch from the facial artery and it runs along the alar groove. The lateral nasal artery also can communicate with the ophthalmic artery, so filler embolus can go to eye and forehead area (**Fig. 5**).

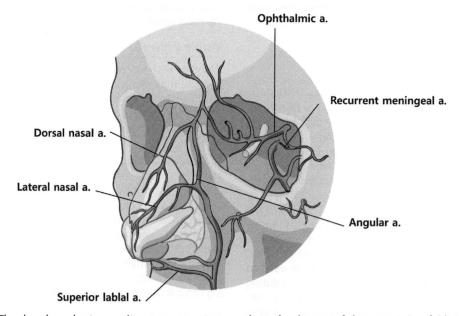

Fig. 5. The dorsal nasal artery, as its name suggests, runs along the dorsum of the nose. It is a fairly immobile blood vessel fixed to the surrounding tissue, and the needle tip can be inserted into the blood vessel if it is inserted in parallel with the blood vessel. The dorsal nasal artery anastomoses with branches of the facial artery so the widespread embolism through the connected blood vessels manifests as skin necrosis in a geographic pattern. It is also a branch of ophthalmic artery, so propagation of the filler embolus may also cause eye symptoms. The lateral nasal artery is a branch from facial artery and it runs along the alar groove. a., artery. (*Adapted from* Moon HJ. Use of fillers in rhinoplasty. Clin Plast Surg 2016;43(1):307–17; with permission.)

Symptoms Intraarterial embolism has a relatively low incidence but its consequences are devastating. When filler is injected into the arterial bloodstream, the patient experiences very severe pain and sometimes complains of a sensation of something spreading out from the injection site. The area supplied by the blood vessel where filler embolism has occurred becomes pale due to ischemia. The ischemic area develops edema within several hours, and soon appears mottled and purplish owing to venous congestion as a rebound phenomenon. After about 24 hours, multiple ulcerative lesions are accompanied by erythema, worsening over time, resulting in desquamation of the tissue. After that, definite findings of dermal necrosis, such as eschar formation, occur gradually. Then the skin recovers through the wound healing process (**Fig. 6**).

Prevention The dorsal nasal artery and the lateral nasal artery are in the superficial fatty layer and SMAS; therefore the injection should be into the deep fatty layer to prevent embolization to the dorsal nasal artery and the lateral nasal artery. Using a blunt cannula also may helpful for beginners who are not familiar with injection technique. If filler must be injected into the side of the nasal dorsum; for example, for correction of deviated nose, the needle should never move in parallel with the direction of the blood vessel. After inserting the needle into the midline, the needle tip should move to the side and inject filler at the same time to prevent injection into the blood vessel, although there may be some bleeding due to injury to the vessel.

Treatment If the patient complains of severe pain and skin turns pale along the area of blood vessel during the filler procedure, stop the injection immediately, and aspirate as much filler as possible. If hyaluronic filler has been injected, injection of hyaluronidase is recommended because

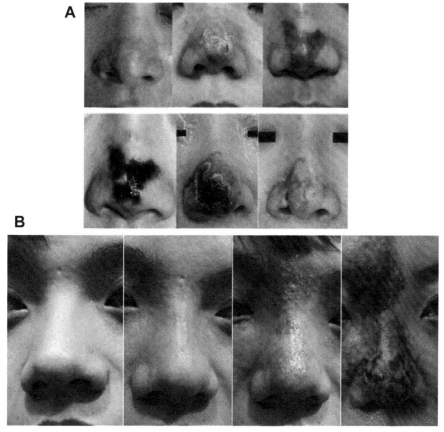

Fig. 6. The ischemic area develops edema within several hours, and soon appears mottled and purplish due to venous congestion as a rebound phenomenon. After about 24 hours, multiple ulcerative lesions, accompanied by erythema, worsen over time, resulting in desquamation of the tissue. After that, definite findings of dermal necrosis, such as eschar formation, occur gradually. Then the skin recovers through the wound healing process. (*A*) Localized type skin necrosis. (*B*) Spreaded type skin necrosis. (*From* Moon HJ. Use of fillers in rhinoplasty. Clin Plast Surg 2016;43(1):307–17; with permission.)

there have been some recent reports that if hyaluronidase is injected around the artery some of it can diffuse through the tunica intima. Some practitioners recommend injection of hyaluronidase regardless of the type of injected filler because hyaluronidase can decrease interstitial pressure.

There are reports that low-molecular-weight heparin therapy decreases thrombosis and embolism; however, it may be difficult to obtain and administer in an outpatient clinic setting. It is very important to supply enough oxygen to the area of ischemia. For this purpose, hot packs and soft massage are applied, and 2% nitroglycerin paste is applied for vasodilation. Starting hyperbaric oxygen therapy is helpful if available. Administer appropriate antibiotics to prevent secondary infection.[20-23] Injection of prostaglandin E1 10 µg a day for 5 days is effective.[24] After about a day, appropriate dressing should be applied after desquamation and pustule formation occur. Apply a wet dressing for faster wound healing and continue to administer antibiotics.

Inflammatory reactions and edema

Sometimes, the protein components such as endotoxin contained in filler may cause inflammatory reactions and edema, and may cause injury in skin. This is caused mostly by hyaluronic acid filler, and symptoms such as erythematous edema, dermal hypertrophy, pustule, and so forth, appear several days after injection.

Symptoms occur at all sites of filler injection and these symptoms are improved easily by the appropriate antibiotic treatment and dressing.

REFERENCES

1. Constantinidis J, Daniilidis J. Aesthetic and functional rhinoplasty. Hosp Med 2005;66:221-6.
2. Murray CA, Zloty D, Warshawski L. The evolution of soft tissue fillers in clinical practice. Dermatol Clin 2005;23:343-63.
3. Oneal RM, Izenberg PH, Schlesinger J. Surgical anatomy of the nose. In: Daniel RK, editor. Rhinoplasty. Boston: Little Brown; 1993. p. 3-37.
4. Daniel RK, Letourneau A. Rhinoplasty: nasal anatomy. Ann Plast Surg 1998;20:5-13.
5. Jung DH, Kim HJ, Koh KS, et al. Arterial supply of the nasal tip in Asians. Laryngoscope 2000; 110(2 Pt 1):308-11.
6. Tardy ME Jr. Pratical surgical anatomy. In: Tardy ME Jr, editor. Rhinoplasty. Philadelphia: W.B. Saunders Co; 1997. p. 5-125.
7. Yun YS, Choi JC, Jung DH. External nasal appearance by Koreans, photo analysis. J Rhinol 1998;5(2):103-7.
8. Gunter JP. Facial analysis for the rhinoplasty patient. Proceedings of the 14th Dallas Rhinoplasty Symposium. Dallas, February 28-March 3, 1997. Southwestern, 1997. p. 45-55.
9. Kim P, Ahn JT. Structured nonsurgical Asian rhinoplasty. Aesthetic Plast Surg 2012;36(3): 698-703.
10. Tanaka Y, Matsuo K, Yuzuriha S. Westernization of the Asian nose by augmentation of the retropositioned anterior nasal spine with an injectable filler. Eplasty 2011;11:e7.
11. Lee YI, Yang HM, Pyeon HJ, et al. Anatomical and histological study of the arterial distribution in the columellar area, and the clinical implications. Surg Radiol Anat 2014;36(7):669-74.
12. Jacovella PF. Use of calcium hydroxylapatite (Radiesse®) for facial augmentation. Clin Interv Aging 2008;3(1):161-74.
13. Lemperle G, Rullan PP, Gauthier-Hazan N. Avoiding and treating dermal filler complications. Plast Reconstr Surg 2006;118(3 Suppl):92S-107S.
14. Narins RS, Jewell M, Rubin M, et al. Clinical conference: management of rare events following dermal fillers - focal necrosis and angry red bumps. Dermatol Surg 2006;32:426-34.
15. Dayan SH, Arkins JP, Brindise R. Soft tissue fillers and biofilms. Facial Plast Surg 2011;27:23-8.
16. Ledon JA, Savas JA, Yang S, et al. Inflammatory nodules following soft tissue filler use: a review of causative agents, pathology and treatment options. Am J Clin Dermatol 2013;14(5):401-11.
17. Kim DW, Yoon ES, Ji YH, et al. Vascular complications of hyaluronic acid fillers and the role of hyaluronidase in management. J Plast Reconstr Aesthet Surg 2011;64(12):1590-5.
18. Cohen JL. Understanding, avoiding, and managing dermal filler complications. Dermatol Surg 2008; 34(Suppl. 1):S92-9.
19. Weinberg MJ, Solish N. Complications of hyaluronic acid fillers. Facial Plast Surg 2009;25:324-8.
20. Grunebaum LD, Allemann IB, Dayan S, et al. The risk of alar necrosis associated with dermal filler injection. Dermatol Surg 2009;35:1635-40.
21. Glaich AS, Cohen JL, Goldberg LH. Injection necrosis of the glabella: protocol for prevention and treatment after use of dermal fillers. Dermatol Surg 2006; 32:276-81.
22. Sclafani AP, Fagien S. Treatment of injectable soft tissue filler complications. Dermatol Surg 2009;35: 1672-80.
23. Hirsch RJ, Lupo M, Cohen JC, et al. Delayed presentation of impending necrosis following soft tissue augmentation with hyaluronic acid and successful management with hyaluronidase. J Drugs Dermatol 2007;6:325-8.
24. Kim SG, Kim YJ, Lee SI, et al. Salvage of nasal skin in a case of venous compromise after hyaluronic acid filler injection using prostaglandin E. Dermatol Surg 2011;37:1817-9.

Septal Extension Graft in Asian Rhinoplasty

Na-Hyun Hwang, MD, MSc, Eun-Sang Dhong, MD, PhD*

KEYWORDS

- Rhinoplasty • Secondary rhinoplasty • Septorhinoplasty • Caudal septal extension
- Extended spreader graft • Septal L-strut extension • Tongue-in-groove

KEY POINTS

- The lower two-thirds of an Asian nose can be enhanced anteriorly and caudally using a septal L-strut extension graft.
- Septal L-strut extension comprises caudal septal extension using a modified tongue-in-groove technique and anterior extended spreader graft.
- The purpose of this technique is to create stability and support to the septum-dependent dorsum, as well as the septum-dependent tip.
- The septal L-strut extension graft is indicated in primary cases in which the bony dorsum is acceptable but the cartilaginous dorsum is relatively hypoplastic.
- In secondary cases, such as an iatrogenic short-nose deformity due to alloplastic implants, the septal L-strut extension graft comprises the autogenous tissue to the dorsum and tip.

Video content accompanies this article at http://www.facialplastic.theclinics.com.

INTRODUCTION AND OVERVIEW

A short nose is among the greatest challenges in rhinoplasty, regardless of patient ethnicity. Direct elongation of the septum resolves the shortness and complements the central nasal area, allowing for the next step on the lateral side of the lower third of the nose. The septal extension graft (SEG) is a method of controlling nasal tip projection, shape, and rotation. In accordance with intended use and quantity of harvested septal cartilage, 3 different types of grafts have been designed: spreader type, batten type, and direct type.[1] However, the unilateral application of the SEG has been criticized because of the potential shift to either side of the caudal septum. Sufficient stability can be obtained with the tongue-and-groove technique.[2] This stabilizes the dorsum

and supplies a platform for the columellar strut, which is then sutured to the bilateral medial crura. This provides stability and support, enabling the SEG to maintain its midline position rather than being distorted to either side.

Since its introduction, the SEG has extensively been the primary choice to correct a small nose and an iatrogenic foreshortened nose, especially in Asian rhinoplasty. However, there are differences in the properties and uses of SEGs in Asian patients. In general, SEGs provide nasal lengthening and tip projection. In Asian rhinoplasty, however, the SEG provides greater projection of the nasal tip. The nasal dorsum needs to be projected anteriorly from nasion to tip in accordance with increased tip projection. Therefore, higher dorsal augmentation is needed for a more harmonious nasal profile after SEG placement in Asian

Disclosure Statement: The authors have nothing to disclose.

Department of Plastic and Reconstructive Surgery, Korea University College of Medicine, Guro Hospital, Korea University Medical Center, 148, Gurodong-ro, Guro-Gu, Seoul 152-703, Republic of Korea

* Corresponding author.

E-mail address: prsdhong@kumc.or.kr

Facial Plast Surg Clin N Am 26 (2018) 331–341
https://doi.org/10.1016/j.fsc.2018.03.007

patients. The problem is that most dorsal augmentation is performed with alloplastic implants in Asian rhinoplasty. The combined use of the SEG and dorsal implant has supplanted other techniques in Asian rhinoplasty (**Fig. 1**).

ALLOPLASTIC IMPLANT WITH COMPLEX ANTERIOR SEPTAL SURGERY

When applying SEGs and spreader grafts, separation of the upper lateral cartilage from the anterior septum is the preferred procedure. Although the mucoperichondrium is well-preserved with full separation from the septal cartilage, even without communication between the dissected pocket and nasal cavity, placing an alloplastic implant on the platform of a widely dissected dorsum may not be safe (see **Fig. 1**). An acute postoperative infection around the implant may spread into the dissected septum, resulting in a disastrous intraseptal abscess. Most patients with severe infection, regardless of acuteness or chronicity, will develop nasal foreshortening due to septal framework and soft tissue destruction. Even when the capsule around the alloplastic implant is safe, the question of longevity remains. Gravity causes alloplastic implants to continuously compress the underlying platform, adding to the pressure exerted from the surrounding soft tissues (**Fig. 2**). Salvage of an infected nose following septorhinoplasty is completely different from salvage of an infected nose following a relatively simple rhinoplasty. In cases of acute or delayed infection, complete extirpation of infectious soft tissue, including the capsule, as well as vigorous irrigation, may salvage the nose if the septum has not been dissected. However, in complex septorhinoplasty cases, even after complete eradication of a septal abscess, loss of nasal support follows, and moderate to severe deformity may remain (**Fig. 3**).

Chronic inflammation with fluctuance can result from compound nasal surgery, which includes complex septal surgery, lateral osteotomy, and dorsal alloplastic implants. Biopsies mostly reveal fluid collection surrounded by a thick capsule with a shiny lining on the inner surface. A bacterial biofilm may rarely initiate intractable chronic infection and cause impending extrusion of alloplastic implants.[3] Ingrowth of synovium-like mucosa or de novo proliferation of the endothelium requires further research (**Fig. 4**). Foreshortening after inflammation closely resembles breast capsular contracture. With severe inflammation, a dense, avascular connective tissue layer forms around the capsule by aggregation of monocytes and fibroblasts. Synovial metaplasia may also play a part in causing contractures.[4]

SPECIFIC CONSIDERATIONS OF SEPTAL EXTENSION GRAFTS IN ASIAN PATIENTS

The septal cartilage in Asian patients tends to be smaller than that in white patients. The mean septal cartilage area in Korean patients is reportedly 8.18 cm^2 to 8.57 cm^2 in men and 7.36 cm^2 in women.[5] The amount of harvested septal cartilage is usually insufficient for multiple simultaneous grafts in Korean patients. Therefore, additional grafts from the concha and costal cartilage should be considered preoperatively.[6] The septal cartilage is thinner in Asian patients, and submucous resection (SMR) of the quadrangular cartilage has a tendency to weaken nasal support. The swing-door procedure performed above the maxillary crest and anterior nasal spine (ANS) for the correction of caudal septal deviation worsens septal instability at the nasal base.[7] Even with a successful bilateral spreader graft, a firm attachment between the ANS and the posterior septal angle is required to provide sufficient support. Furthermore, in Asian patients, in whom the middle and medial crura are relatively weak, overcoming a weakened nasal base is the greatest obstacle in obtaining a stable tip. Most Asian rhinoplasties require 2 different dimensional enhancements: anteroposterior and cephalocaudal lengthening. When the nasal length is extended, the height of the nasal dorsum must often be increased. Many

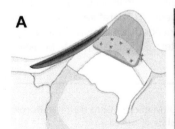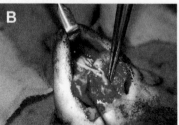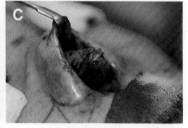

Fig. 1. SEG and insertion of an alloplastic implant. (*A*) This schematic shows the most popular technique performed in Asian patients. (*B*) Creating a flat platform by applying a complex SEG. (*C*) Dorsal augmentation with a silicone implant following SEG.

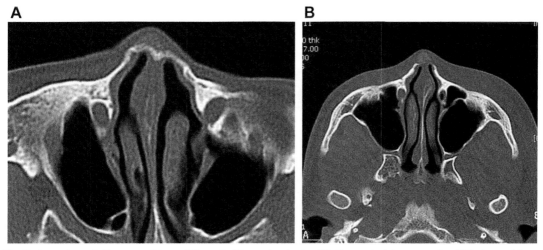

Fig. 2. Long-term follow-up of two different silicone implants. (*A*) Computed tomography (CT) showed bony resorption beneath the 4-mm-thick silicone implant in a 50-year-old woman. The implant was inserted 14 years prior and osteotomies were not performed. (*B*) A 32-year-old woman reported pain of the dorsum 5 years postoperatively, and CT revealed resorption at the keystone area.

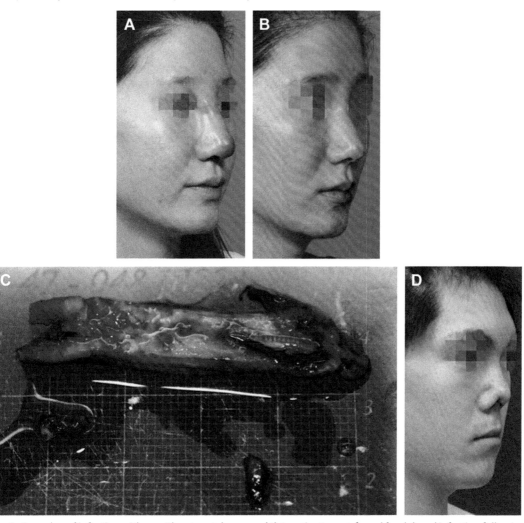

Fig. 3. Sequelae of infection with or without septal surgery. (*A*) A patient was referred for delayed infection following silicone implantation without septal surgery 5 years prior. (*B*) The nose was salvaged without severe sequelae after total extirpation of the capsule and infected soft tissue. (*C*) Excised capsule around the silicone implant. (*D*) A patient with a severely contracted nose and tip who had undergone surgery (with septal surgery) similar to that shown in **Fig. 1**.

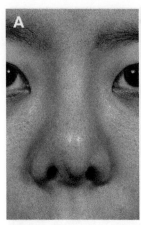
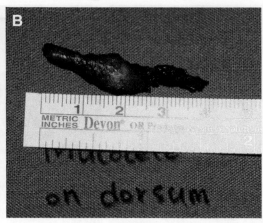
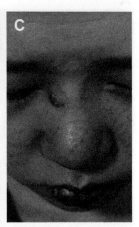

Fig. 4. Various features of mucocele-like capsules. (*A*) A patient showed impending silicone extrusion and discoloration of the tip. (*B*) The capsule was filled with fluid and the inner lining was covered by a synovium-like membrane. (*C*) A patient who was referred with the diagnosis of epidermal cyst. A mucocele-like capsule was totally excised using open rhinoplasty.

investigators have reported various methods and designs to overcome the smaller Asian septal cartilage.[8–12] However, most of these only involve limited applications in the cephalocaudal direction. Dorsal augmentation must also be carefully considered. It is self-contradictory to treat the nasal contracture caused by an alloplastic implant with another alloplastic implant in the nasal dorsum.

CLINICAL FEATURES OF THE ASIAN FACE FROM THE LATERAL VIEW

In the sagittal view, the dorsum can be classified into the bony dorsum and cartilaginous dorsum. There are 4 possible combinations in this classification, depending on whether the nasal bone and nasion anterior projection is high or low, and whether the septal portion is high or low. Developmentally, the bony dorsum and cartilaginous dorsum develop together; thus, a low bony dorsum with a high cartilaginous dorsum is rarely seen.

HIGH BONY DORSUM WITH HIGH CARTILAGINOUS DORSUM

This is managed with reduction rhinoplasty and represents cases for which Asian rhinoplasty and Western operations are similar. The goal is to create a balance between the locations of the hump and tip to achieve a dorsal esthetic line. Normally, medial and lateral osteotomies are also performed, and dorsal onlay grafts are not necessary, except in cases of a very low nasion. A larger hump requires more spreader graft use because removal of large lesions leads to an increased

likelihood of nasal airway obstruction after removal (**Fig. 5**, upper row).

ACCEPTABLE BONY DORSUM WITH UNDERDEVELOPED CARTILAGINOUS DORSUM

This corresponds to a mild nasal hump, saddle nose, and underprojected tip. Extended camouflage leads to increased height of the bony dorsum, causing disruption of the dorsal esthetic line. In this case, it is more harmonious to only perform anterior projection of the cartilaginous dorsum, according to the ideal tip projection. If the entire length of the nose is augmented for dorsal camouflage of the lower two-thirds, the bony dorsum becomes too high. Thus, it is more appropriate to perform anterior extension and accompanying caudal extension of the remaining septum without touching the bony dorsum. The septal L-strut extension, introduced in this article, is the most effective method (see **Fig. 5**, middle row).

PRIMARY SMALL NOSE

In a patient with a low profile in all areas of the nose, including the nasion, the bony dorsum and cartilaginous dorsum are equally low. It is rare to see septal deviation in a small nose. A primary short nose has insufficient length and quantity, even with a massive SMR, because it yields a relatively small septal cartilage. In a primary case in which intranasal inspection reveals a very weak septal cartilage, septorhinoplasty is least indicated because an SMR can lead to even weaker nasal support. Instead, it is wiser to perform a camouflage method with a dorsal onlay graft and tip

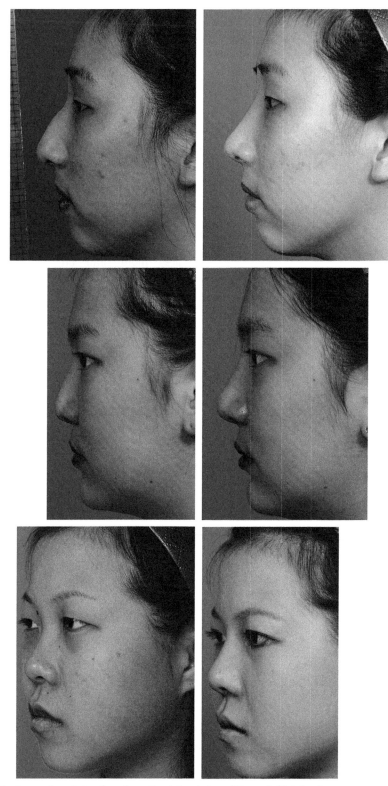

Fig. 5. Clinical features of an Asian face from the lateral view. (*Upper left*) Asian hump nose, preoperative view. (*Upper right*) Asian hump nose, postoperative view. The operative technique is the same as in Western patients. (*Middle left*) A patient in whom the bony dorsum was fairly high but the lower two-thirds was hypoplastic and underprojected. (*Middle right*) The septal L-strut was extended anteriorly and caudally. (*Lower left*) A patient with a small nose, showing a low nasal dorsum, underprojected tip, and short nose. (*Lower right*) The dorsum was augmented with a silicone implant and tip plasty was performed using a columellar strut and cartilage graft.

plasty. Because the amount of cartilage is insufficient, concha or rib cartilage can be used for septal reconstruction and extension; however, it is safer to perform autografts in the dorsum (see **Fig. 5**, lower row).

SECONDARY CONTRACTED NOSE

This is the most common iatrogenic complication in Asian septorhinoplasties and the most difficult to correct esthetically. In a secondary case, greater midline elongation is needed compared with a primary case. Because strong support is needed to overcome the infection-induced shortening of the skin and soft tissue envelope, septal reconstruction with septal extension is necessary.

TECHNIQUES OF SEPTAL L-STRUT EXTENSION GRAFT IN ASIAN PATIENTS

An effective L-strut (anterocaudal) extension requires various combinations of autologous cartilage. Sometimes it is impossible to perform an effective L-strut extension with only the septal cartilage due to insufficient quantity. To perform an L-strut extension with only autologous tissue, cymba concha or cavum concha cartilage is required, and rib cartilage is needed if the concha cartilage has already been used. In patients with small ears, rib cartilage can be chosen as the primary option.

CAUDAL SEPTAL EXTENSION: MODIFIED TONGUE-IN-GROOVE TECHNIQUE

Because using the septal cartilage in the support line of the anterior portion is more advantageous in obtaining a straight dorsal profile, other cartilage must often be used caudally. For caudal L-strut extension, rib cartilage provides the most plentiful source if septal cartilage is insufficient; however, considering its stiffness, it is most advantageous to use cymba concha cartilage in Asian patients. In the senior author's 15 years of experience, the cymba concha has been used on the caudal septum for modified tongue-in-groove technique and has been useful in obtaining tip projection. The cymba concha, when folded, can yield more than 7 mm width and 20 mm length, and is adequate to support the middle and medial crura of the lower lateral cartilage in Asian patients (**Fig. 6**A).[13] In particular, if the tongue-in-groove technique is applied at the ANS using the cymba concha to correct the loss of tip support after performing a caudal septal swing-door technique, it is possible to achieve both projection and stability. Additional support can be obtained by suturing with the concave sides facing each other during folding. It is also important to attach the perichondrium of the cymba concha to obtain additional strength from the brittle concha (**Fig. 6**B).

EXTENDED SPREADER GRAFT: ANTEROCAUDAL EXTENSION

Septal cartilage is most suitable for L-strut anterior extension. Anterior extension requires more width than other spreader grafts. This can be described as a visible spreader graft. As anterior extension is possible from the keystone area to the tip, excessive anterior extension must be avoided, because it leads to difficulty in obtaining a smooth line in the keystone area and requires more graft on the nasion. Multiple sutures are needed between the anterior margin of the existing septum and posterior margin of the inserted extended spreader graft (**Fig. 6**C) (Video 1).

CAMOUFLAGE GRAFT AT RADIX AREA

L-strut anterior extension often requires an onlay graft of the radix area for smoothness and for the dorsal aesthetic line. The starting point of the nose can be augmented using various types of grafts: dermis from the midsacral area, fascia from deep temporalis muscle, superficial mastoid fascia,[14] and diced cartilage with fascia. For the correction of an irregular surface at the nasal bone and cartilage junction, a thin layer of soft tissue graft is helpful (**Fig. 6**D).

CREATING AN ANTERIOR SEPTAL ANGLE AND RAFTING GRAFT

After the anterior angle of the 2 extensions is approximated, a new anterior septal angle is established. Usually, 4 layers of cartilage are sutured at this area to create a new anterior septal angle. If there is instability with the anterior and caudal struts, a small piece of cartilage can be applied as a rafter for reinforcement (**Fig. 6**E).

RELOCATING THE LOWER LATERAL CARTILAGE

After L-strut extension is performed, the new position of the middle crura will be a new tip-defining point. Various sutures, including an interdomal suture, intercrural suture, and lateral crura-spanning suture, are indispensable for tip complex positioning. The cartilaginous dorsum and tip are septum-dependent.

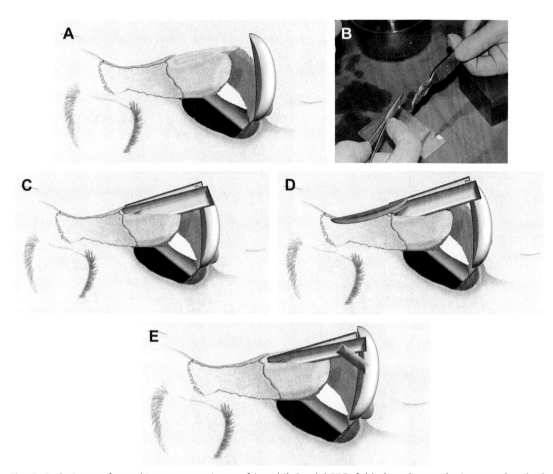

Fig. 6. Techniques of septal L-strut extension grafting. (*A*) Caudal SEG: folded cymba concha is sutured on both sides of the ANS for support and caudal extension, a modified tongue-in-groove technique. (*B*) Folded cymba concha: facing concave sides were sutured. Minimal continuity in the middle enhances strength. (*C*) Bilateral extended spreader graft: visible spreader grafts are applied anteriorly. (*D*) Radix graft: any type of soft tissue is grafted on the nasion to smooth the dorsum. (*E*) Rafting graft: small pieces of cartilage are applied between the anterior and caudal pillars.

SEPTAL L-STRUT EXTENSION IN PRIMARY SEPTORHINOPLASTY
Indications

Septal L-strut extension technique is primarily indicated for a mild nasal hump, saddle nose, or nose with an underprojected lower two-thirds and deviated septum.

Pitfalls

- The amount of quadrangular cartilage harvested from a small nose is relatively small.
- Proper length of the spreader graft cannot be achieved with a severely deformed septal cartilage.

Case 1

A 27-year-old woman was referred for the correction of a deviated nose. She had symptoms of nasal obstruction (Nasal Obstruction Symptom Evaluation [NOSE] score: 10), and wanted a straighter nose and more projected tip. The donor sites were the right cymba and cavum concha and the septal quadrangular cartilage (**Fig. 7**).

Case 2

A 22-year-old man with a saddle nose and mild hump was referred for septorhinoplasty. He had mild nasal obstruction on the left (NOSE score: 7), and wanted the tip and dorsum enhanced. He did not want a higher nasal root. Right cymba concha was harvested and folded for the caudal SEG and a new anterior septal angle was created using the septal L-strut extension graft (**Fig. 8**).

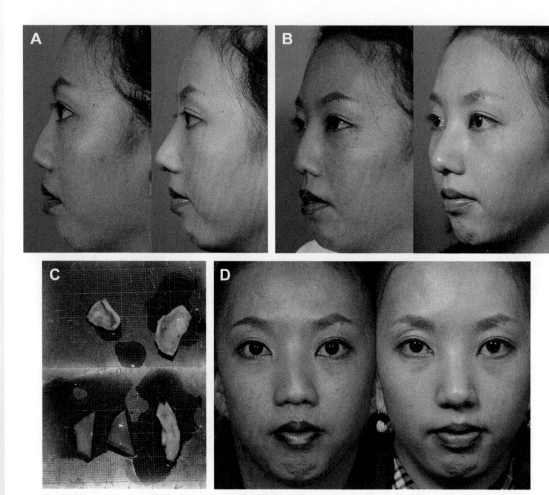

Fig. 7. Case 1: A patient with deviated nose and tip underprojection. (*A*) Lateral view: (*left*) preoperative view, (*right*) postoperative 1 year. (*B*) Quarter view. (*C*) Cavum (*above*) and cymba concha (*below*): very thin and weak septal cartilage was divided and the cymba concha was folded. (*D*) Frontal view.

SEPTAL L-STRUT EXTENSION IN SECONDARY SEPTORHINOPLASTY

Indications

This technique is best for iatrogenic short-nose deformity due to previous alloplastic implants and saddle-nose deformity after SMR. Patients who have previously received implants have strong antipathy for another implant.

Pitfalls

- An appropriate amount of autologous cartilage should be prepared. In most secondary cases, septal and concha cartilages may no longer exist. Rib cartilage is the best and final source for septal reconstruction.[15]
- The septal L-strut extension graft can be applied using folded cymba concha and folded cavum concha in most Asian patients (**Fig. 9**).
- Dissecting the septum may be impossible in cases in which the mucoperichondrium has been destroyed.
- Severe destruction can occur where porous polyethylene material is applied at the septum as a spreader or SEG.
- If there is severe destruction at the keystone area, stable fixation between the caudal nasal bone and anterior grafts is needed after drill holes are made. The same principle applies for the ANS area.

Case 3

A 38-year-old woman was referred for contracture and upward malposition of a preexisting L-type silicone implant; she wanted to correct the short-nose deformity. The implant was removed and a septal L-strut extension procedure was

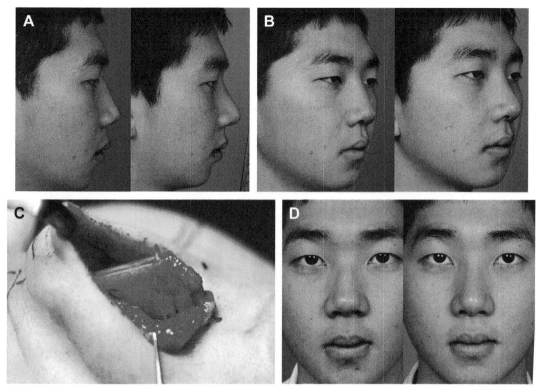

Fig. 8. Case 2: A patient with mild hump and saddle-nose deformity. (*A*) Lateral view: (*left*) preoperative view, (*right*) postoperative 1 month. (*B*) Quarter view. (*C*) Creation of a new anterior septal angle by suturing the anterior and caudal pillars. (*D*) Frontal view.

performed using her left seventh rib. Rectus abdominis fascia was harvested and applied as an onlay graft to smooth the dorsal profile (**Fig. 10**).

Case 4

A 53-year-old man was referred for a severe saddle-nose deformity. Both cymba and cavum conchae were applied for the L-strut extension.

The dorsum was grafted using right superficial mastoid fascia (**Fig. 11**).

COMPLICATIONS

The same complications that affect conventional SEGs occur in the L-strut extension graft: stiffness, decreased projection, nasal tip deviation, and infection. However, L-strut extension has a great advantage compared with autologous-only

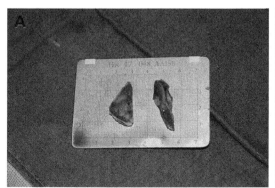

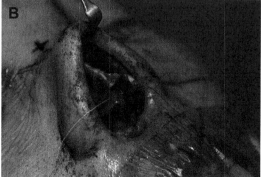

Fig. 9. L-strut extension using cymba and cavum conchae. (*A*) (*Left*) folded cavum concha, (*right*) folded cymba concha. (*B*) The L-strut was reconstructed using dorsal cavum concha and caudal cymba concha.

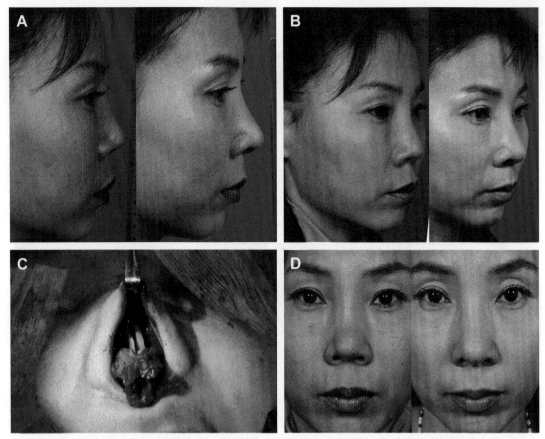

Fig. 10. Case 3: A patient with iatrogenic foreshortened nose. (*A*) Lateral view: (*left*) preoperative view, (*right*) postoperative 3 months. (*B*) Quarter view. (*C*) After L-type silicone was removed, the septal L-strut was reconstructed with sliced rib cartilage. (*D*) Frontal view.

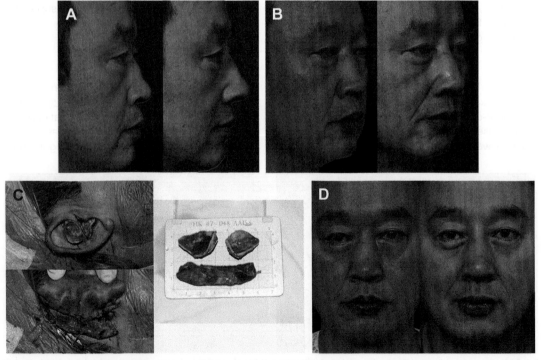

Fig. 11. Case 4: A patient with severe saddle-nose deformity. (*A*) Lateral view: (*left*) preoperative view, (*right*) postoperative 6 months. (*B*) Quarter view. (*C*) Cavum concha and cymba concha autografts were used in making the L-strut and superficial mastoid fascia was grafted on the dorsum. (*D*) Frontal view.

techniques in dealing with the relatively small Asian septorhinoplasty.

SUMMARY

The septal L-strut extension graft is useful in augmenting the lower two-thirds of the nose anteriorly and caudally in relatively small Asian noses. The septal L-strut extension comprises a caudally extended septal batten graft and anteriorly extended spreader graft. The purpose of this technique is to create a septum-dependent dorsum, as well as a septum-dependent tip. Consequently, the need to apply alloplastic implants may be reduced.

SUPPLEMENTARY DATA

Supplementary data related to this article can be found online at https://doi.org/10.1016/j.fsc.2018.03.007.

REFERENCES

1. Byrd HS, Andochick S, Copit S, et al. Septal extension grafts: a method of controlling tip projection shape. Plast Reconstr Surg 1997;100(4):999–1010.
2. Guyuron B, Varghai A. Lengthening the nose with a tongue-and-groove technique. Plast Reconstr Surg 2003;111(4):1533–9 [discussion: 1540–1].
3. Walker TJ, Toriumi DM. Analysis of facial implants for bacterial biofilm formation using scanning electron microscopy. JAMA Facial Plast Surg 2016;18(4):299–304.
4. Siggelkow W, Faridi A, Spiritus K, et al. Histological analysis of silicone breast implant capsules and correlation with capsular contracture. Biomaterials 2003;24(6):1101–9.
5. Hwang SM, Lim O, Hwang MK, et al. The clinical analysis of the nasal septal cartilage by measurement using computed tomography. Arch Craniofac Surg 2016;17(3):140–5.
6. Kim JS, Khan NA, Song HM, et al. Intraoperative measurements of harvestable septal cartilage in rhinoplasty. Ann Plast Surg 2010;65(6):519–23.
7. Dhong ES. Septorhinoplasty: endoscopic approach and reinforcement of nasal support line. J Korean Soc Aesthetic Plast Surg 2010;16(3):111–6.
8. Huang J, Liu Y. A modified technique of septal extension using a septal cartilage graft for short-nose rhinoplasty in Asians. Aesthetic Plast Surg 2012;36(5):1028–38.
9. Zelken J, Chang CS, Chuang SS, et al. An economical approach to ethnic Asian rhinoplasty. Facial Plast Surg 2016;32(1):95–104.
10. Woo JS, Dung NP, Suh MK. A novel technique for short nose correction: hybrid septal extension graft. J Craniofac Surg 2016;27(1):e44–8.
11. Dhong ES, Kim YJ, Suh MK. L-shaped columellar strut in East Asian nasal tip plasty. Arch Plast Surg 2013;40(5):616–20.
12. Chang YL. Correction of difficult short nose by modified caudal septal advancement in Asian patients. Aesthet Surg J 2010;30(2):166–75.
13. Dhong ES, Han SK, Lee CH, et al. Anthropometric study of alar cartilage in Asians. Ann Plast Surg 2002;48(4):386–91.
14. Hong ST, Kim DW, Yoon ES, et al. Superficial mastoid fascia as an accessible donor for various augmentations in Asian rhinoplasty. J Plast Reconstr Aesthet Surg 2012;65(8):1035–40.
15. Toriumi DM, Pero CD. Asian rhinoplasty. Clin Plast Surg 2010;37(2):335–52.

Tip Grafting for the Asian Nose

Yong Ju Jang, MD, PhD[a],*, Sung Hee Kim, MD[b]

KEYWORDS

- Asian rhinoplasty • Tip grafting • Tip onlay graft • Shield graft • Multilayer tip grafting

KEY POINTS

- Asian noses tend to have a weak cartilage framework, thick skin, and abundant soft tissue; major tip refinement with tip grafts is required to create more tip projection and definition.
- The best tip refinement approach in patients with thick skin and poorly developed tip cartilage is tip grafting with thick and rigid costal cartilage.
- The most important grafting techniques are tip onlay graft, shield graft, and multilayer tip graft.
- We classified Korean noses into 4 classes based on their alar cartilage shape and specify grafting procedures that will generate an acceptable tip in these different tip shapes.
- Because Asians vary in their cartilage configuration, skin thickness, and aesthetic desires, a tailored tip grafting strategy is needed to meet the aesthetic goal of the individual patient.

 Video content accompanies this article at http://www.facialplastic.theclinics.com.

INTRODUCTION

Techniques for surgical refinement of the nasal tip include resection or division of the lower lateral cartilage,[1–3] suturing of the lower lateral cartilage,[3] and cartilage grafting.[4] The latter 2 techniques are particularly commonly used for tip refinement.

Asian noses tend to have a weak cartilage framework, thick skin, and abundant soft tissue that yield a less refined nasal dorsum and tip.[5] These anatomic features mean that tip surgery is the most difficult part of rhinoplasty in Asian patients. The thickness of the nasal skin in particular plays an important role in the success of tip refinement techniques. We previously reported that Koreans have thicker nasal skin than Caucasians.[6] Specifically, Korean nasal skin is thickest over the nasofrontal angle, becomes thinner over the rhinion, thickens again at the nasal tip, and then thins over the columella. We observed that thicker skin at the nasal tip and columella is associated with poor tip refinement outcomes. Thus, regional skin thickness may be an important prognostic factor for the success of tip surgery.

Although the tip suture technique can effectively improve the shape of the nasal tip in subjects with relatively well-developed lower lateral cartilage and thin skin,[7,8] it often does not provide sufficient tip projection in Asian noses when it is used on its own. By contrast, tip grafting can effectively improve the tip projection, rotation, and definition in Asian noses because it is less affected by skin thickness than the tip suture technique.[5] As a result, we mostly use the tip grafting technique to refine the tip of Asian noses. Herein, we discuss the most common types of tip graft materials, the

Disclosure Statement: The authors have nothing to disclose.
[a] Department of Otolaryngology, Asan Medical Centre, University of Ulsan College of Medicine, 88 Olympic-ro 43-gil, Songpa-gu, Seoul 05505, Republic of Korea; [b] Department of Otolaryngology, National Medical Centre, Seoul, Republic of Korea
* Corresponding author.
E-mail address: jangyj@amc.seoul.kr

Facial Plast Surg Clin N Am 26 (2018) 343–356
https://doi.org/10.1016/j.fsc.2018.03.008

various tip grafting methods, and which of these methods is best suited for specific tip shapes. The complications that can arise after tip grafting and how to manage them are also discussed.

TIP GRAFTING MATERIALS

The most important factors when selecting the material for tip grafting are the quantity and quality of the available cartilage and the thickness of the skin.

Septal Cartilage

If there is sufficient septal cartilage with reasonable thickness and rigidity, tip grafting with this material is readily performed. In fact, this tip grafting material is ideal because it obviates the additional morbidity associated with obtaining cartilage from the ear or chest. However, in Asians, the quantity and quality of the septal cartilage are often very limited.[9] This finding is particularly true for female East Asian patients; in these patients, the rhinoplasty surgeon often encounters extremely thin and weak cartilage that cannot bear the weight and tension of the skin that covers the graft. As a result, the nose tip loses its grafted shape after the skin is closed (**Fig. 1**). Furthermore, when tip surgery using weak septal cartilage is performed on patients with thick skin, the grafted cartilage only adds

volume to the tip. Thus, rather than promoting tip projection and definition, the surgery increases tip bulbosity. Consequently, the definition of the tip worsens after closing the skin. Another factor that hampers the use of septal cartilage for tip work is that the thin septal cartilage graft is easily lacerated by the suture material when the graft is fixed via sutures to the underlying lower lateral cartilages.

Conchal Cartilage

When using conchal cartilage for tip surgery, it is desirable to harvest it with the perichondrium attached to both sides, or at least on 1 side.[10] This is because the perichondrium around the cartilage facilitates the suture-induced fixation of the tip graft to the lower lateral cartilage. Moreover, the support from the perichondrium adds to the strength of the conchal cartilage. It should be noted that the conchal cartilage has a natural curvature. The surgeon should ensure that this curvature does not influence the surgical results. If the intrinsic curvature of the conchal cartilage does hamper the achievement of the desired tip shape, a few cross-hatched incisions can eliminate the curvature. However, the natural curvature of the conchal cartilage can also be exploited in shield grafting (discussed elsewhere in this article); when the shield-shaped conchal cartilage is placed in the nasal tip lobule with its concave side facing the caudal direction, it can improve tip definition while preventing cephalic bending of the tip graft. This technique is especially useful in patients with thick skin (**Fig. 2**). When considering conchal cartilage for tip grafting, the surgeon must carefully consider the possibility of donor site complications such as hematoma and keloid formation.[11] The latter complication is particularly

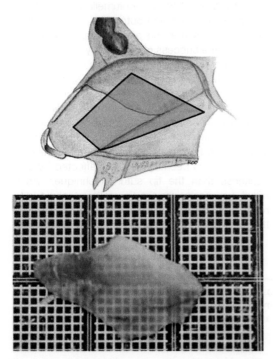

Fig. 1. Thin and weak septal cartilage that is not suitable for tip grafting.

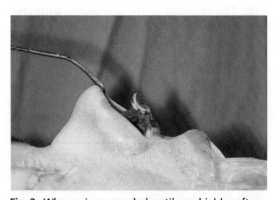

Fig. 2. When using a conchal cartilage shield graft, cephalic bending of the tip graft can be prevented by ensuring that the concave part of the cartilage faces the caudal direction.

concerning because ear keloids are relatively common (1%), they are more likely to develop when conchal cartilage is harvested from the posterior approach, and they are difficult to manage effectively.

Costal Cartilage

In patients with extremely thick skin, septal cartilage or conchal cartilage may not be suitable for tip grafting because they cannot impose marked changes that show through the thick nasal skin–soft tissue envelope. Hence, when a patient with thick skin and poorly developed tip cartilage wants a significant change in their tip shape, it is best to perform tip grafting with thick and rigid costal cartilage after stabilizing the base with a columellar strut or a septal extension graft.[12] Costal cartilage is usually harvested from the 6th or 7th rib, and is cut into several slices by using a dermatome blade. The sliced cartilage pieces can then be shaped further to become a spreader graft, a septal extension graft, a dorsal implant, and/or tip grafts (**Fig. 3**). It is best to harvest the costal cartilage with the perichondrium because the perichondrium can help to camouflage the tip graft. For dorsal augmentation using costal cartilage, the core portion is preferred. By contrast, in tip surgery, both the core and peripheral portions can be used because warping of the cartilage is not an important issue in tip surgery. Despite these advantages, using costal cartilage for tip grafts entails a few difficulties. First, because this cartilage is harder than other cartilages, it is more difficult to suture to the underlying alar cartilage. Moreover, more suture material must be used compared with when other cartilage types are used. This factor is significant because using large amounts of suture material can increase the risk of suture material-related inflammation. Second, in our experience, when large amounts of thick and hard costal cartilage are grafted on the tip, there is a risk that the core

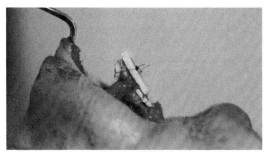

Fig. 3. The harvested costal cartilage is designed into a spreader graft, a dorsal graft, and a tip graft.

portions of these cartilages are not nourished well enough. This lack can lead to necrosis and secondary infections.[13,14] This problem is particularly common when the nose has undergone multiple revisions. This is because these noses often bear considerable scarring and fibrosis that can severely impair the circulation in the nasal skin–soft tissue envelope.

SPECIFIC TIP GRAFTING TECHNIQUES

Various tip grafting techniques have been described. The choice of one over the others should be based on a thoughtful consideration of the desired tip shape, the quality and quantity of available cartilage, and the patient's native tip shape.

Columellar Strut Graft

This technique involves carving a long piece of cartilage into a strut and positioning it between the middle and medial crura of both sides of the lower lateral cartilages. This technique can enhance nasal tip support, provide a moderate degree of tip projection, alter the nostril shape, improve symmetry, and alter the columellar lobular angle.[15] However, we believe that, on its own, the columellar strut cannot fundamentally change the shape of the tip cartilage. Therefore, this technique should only be used to generate a stable foundation for other tip grafts, such as the shield graft or onlay graft. One problem with the columellar strut is that, if it is not properly placed, it may induce cephalic rotation of the tip or columellar deviation. Septal cartilage and costal cartilage are suitable materials for columellar strut grafting. The intrinsic curvature of conchal cartilage does complicate its use as a columellar strut graft. However, if options other than ear cartilage are not available, 2 layers of conchal cartilage that are sewn side by side can serve as a columellar strut graft.

Shield Graft, Also Known as Infratip Lobular Graft

This graft is placed on the middle and medial crura of the lower lateral cartilages. This technique can increase tip projection, improve tip definition, and make the infratip lobule more distinct (**Fig. 4**). If the graft is long, it will not only increase tip projection, it will increase the overall length of the columella. Notably, however, if the graft is short and is placed on the infratip lobule portion, it may bend in the cephalic direction, thereby causing the nasal tip to rotate in the cephalic direction (**Fig. 5**). If the alar

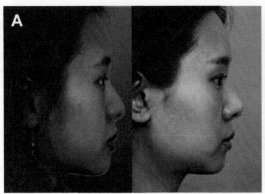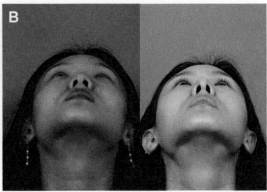

Fig. 4. A patient with a favorable aesthetic change in the nasal tip after shield grafting. Lateral views (*A*) and basal views (*B*).

cartilage exhibits adequate domal angulation, placement of a single shield graft can increase tip projection. However, in patients with round tip cartilage and poor projection, a shield graft will emphasize the round contour rather than improving tip definition. Therefore, in such patients, it may be necessary to place more than 1 layer of shield grafts (multilayer tip grafting, discussed elsewhere in this article).[16] While carving the graft, the graft periphery should be carefully beveled or the cartilage margin should be crushed gently; this step will ensure that the graft margin is not visible through the skin. This margin-trimming procedure is particularly important for patients with thin skin. Shield grafts are usually designed in a shield or ginkgo leaf shape. The top of the graft must be broad so that both ends of the top side can provide tip defining points. Although the leading edge of the shield graft must be slightly higher than the height of the existing dome of the tip, this shape can lead to problematic outcomes

when the nasal skin is thick. This is because it is difficult to obtain cartilage that is strong enough to push up the thick skin that covers the graft. As a result, when the insufficiently strong shield graft is placed and its upper margin is even slightly higher than the dome, it can be bent by the weight of the thick skin, resulting in cephalic bending and an upturned appearance of the nose. To prevent this unwelcome effect, and to reach the desired aesthetic goal, the following techniques can be used (**Fig. 6**).[17] First, a graft that supports the shield from the back of the shield graft can be placed: these are known as cartilage backstops, backing grafts, or buttress grafts. Second, the shield graft can be supported on both sides with a lateral crural onlay graft (discussed elsewhere in this article). Third, a long columellar strut or septal extension graft that is exposed on the top of the dome can be placed to support the shield graft from behind. Fourth, conchal cartilage is used to generate the shield graft and is placed such that its concave surface faces the caudal direction; this causes the graft to exert a springlike force that counteracts the cephalic bending induced by the thick skin (see **Fig. 2**).

The placement of a shield graft can make the nose look longer. Therefore, the shield grafting technique is not advisable in patients with a ptotic tip and dorsal convexity where the nose already looks long. The most notable complication of this technique is an obvious tip graft contour that is visible through the skin. This complication is particularly common in thin-skinned individuals. To prevent this complication, it may be necessary to cover the graft with soft tissues such as fascia or perichondrium. Another possible complication of the shield graft is migration and resultant tip deformity.

Fig. 5. A short shield graft in patients with a round tip cartilage contour may make the nose tip look more rotated.

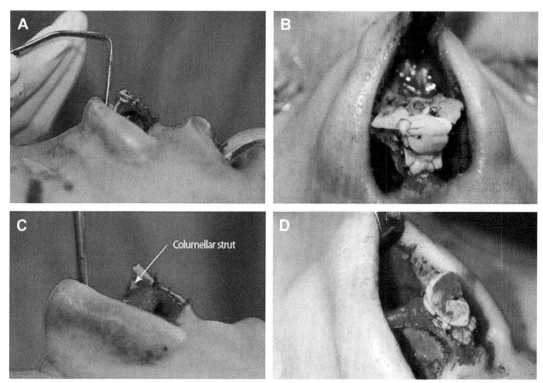

Fig. 6. Different ways of preventing shield grafts from bending in the cephalic direction. (*A*) Placement of a supportive graft behind the shield graft. (*B*) Placement of a lateral crural onlay graft that supports the shield graft on both sides. (*C*) Placement of a columellar strut that is exposed above the dome and thereby supports the shield graft. (*D*) Using conchal cartilage for the shield graft and placing it so that its concave surface faces the caudal direction and thereby exerts a springlike action that counters the cephalic bending of the graft.

Tip Onlay Graft

Unlike the vertically oriented shield graft, tip onlay grafting involves placing 1 or several layers of graft horizontally at the dome of the tip.[4] The width of the onlay graft is greater than its length and height, and it usually has a rectangular shape. This graft must be fixed on the caudal margin of the dome. It softens the transition on the side from the dome to the alar lobule, increases tip projection, and improves definition. In patients with adequate tip support and a certain degree of projection, it can not only increase tip projection, it can also camouflage tip irregularities (**Fig. 7**). If the tip onlay graft is too round and blunt, onlay grafting may not lead to an aesthetically pleasing result (**Fig. 8**). Tip onlay grafting can involve stacking layers of cartilage on top of each other (ie, stacked onlay grafting). However, although this can improve tip projection to some extent when the tip is viewed from the lateral side, it can also make the infratip lobule seem unnaturally long when viewed from the basal side. Visible graft contour is also a common complication of the tip onlay graft. Tip onlay grafting is ideal for creating a natural-looking supratip break; this procedure is particularly suitable for patients with a convex nasal dorsum.

Multilayer (Multitier) Cartilaginous Tip Graft

Often, a desired tip shape with good definition and projection cannot be obtained by simply placing a shield graft or a tip onlay graft. This is because an underprojected tip often presents with a round tip contour that is worsened when a single shield graft or onlay graft layer is placed. Therefore, to create the desired tip contour with the ideal vectors of projection, several layers of cartilage must be placed (**Fig. 9**).[16] The concept is analogous to creating a hill on the top of a mountain or adding a second tip. This technique is also useful for elongating the central compartment of the nose in patients with a short nose (**Fig. 10**). This procedure has some distinct advantages. First, it is a very flexible approach that can be tailored to suit the shapes and configurations of the lower lateral cartilages and it results in an aesthetically pleasing tip shape without unwanted cephalic rotation. Second, it yields good tip definition in patients with thick skin. However,

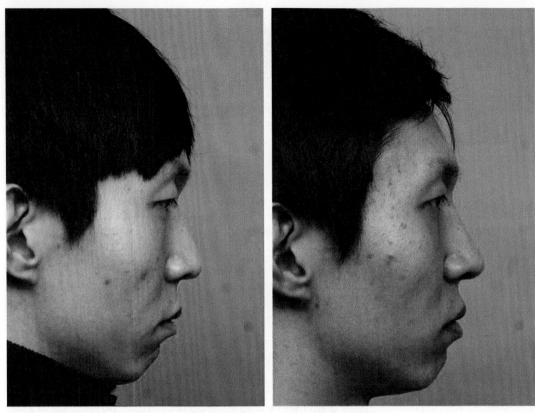

Fig. 7. A patient with an improved tip shape as a result of tip onlay grafting.

multilayer cartilaginous tip grafting does have some potential drawbacks. First, a relatively large amount of cartilage is needed to generate the tip framework. Hence, the procedure may be associated with donor site morbidity. Second, there is a relatively high risk of tip graft visibility after surgery. Third, the use of multiple cartilage grafts may increase the risk of inflammation and secondary infection.

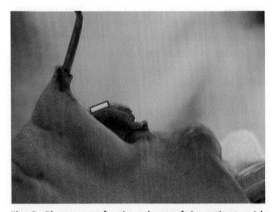

Fig. 8. Placement of a tip onlay graft in patients with a round tip contour cannot generate an ideal tip contour.

Multilayer tip grafting is usually conducted via an external approach. Thus, depending on the amount of cartilage that is required, septal, conchal, tragal, and/or costal cartilage are harvested. Depending on the number of layers that are needed, the cartilage is cut into multiple shield-shaped grafts, each of which is shorter than the preceding graft but approximately the same width. If necessary, caudal extension of the septum, columellar strut placement, and dome suturing is performed before the multilayer tip graft is placed. In multilayer tip grafting, the first layer, which is the longest of the cut grafts, is placed at the caudal aspect of the middle and medial crus and secured with 5-0 polydioxanone sutures such that its leading (superior) edge is higher than the height of the existing dome. The subsequent layer, which is the next longest graft, is placed centrally on top of the first graft so that its superior edge is higher than the first graft (Video 1). The next grafts, if used, are placed in the same manner. The number of graft layers used depends on how much projection is required and is determined intraoperatively. In most cases, we prefer to place only 2 graft layers. We find that the first layer achieves the desired tip projection and the second layer provides

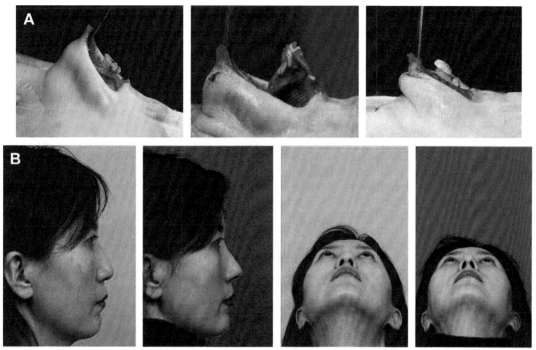

Fig. 9. Various form of multilayer tip grafting technique (*A*). Typical patient showing improved tip aesthetics after multilayer tip graft (*B*).

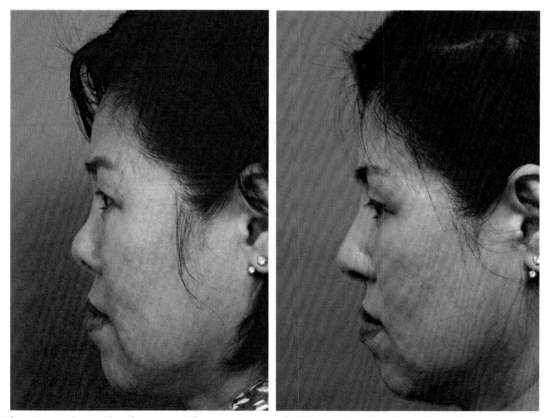

Fig. 10. A patient with a short nose deformity was treated with a combination of an extended spreader graft, a caudal septal extension graft, dorsal augmentation, and multilayer tip grafting.

additional projection and a natural-looking infratip break (**Fig. 11**). When performing 2-layer grafting, the second layer of graft should have a wide top and a narrower bottom. However, the horizontal width of the most caudally located graft depends on the thickness of the tip skin. For thin skin, a larger horizontal width will provide smooth tip definition. For thick skin, a narrower width can result in better aesthetic results. To provide an aesthetically pleasing tip contour, it is important to meticulously smooth the graft margins by gentle carving. Cephalic bending of the tip grafts can be prevented by placing a conchal cartilage graft such that its concave surface faces the caudal direction. A backing graft may also be needed to prevent cephalic bending of the grafts. If the tip grafts are too conspicuous (a phenomenon that is more likely to occur in patients with thin tip skin), perichondrium, fascia, or crushed cartilage can be placed to smooth the graft edges.

Modified Vertical Dome Division Technique

The classical vertical dome division involves excising the dome, including the skin, medializing it, and sewing it together at the midline. Although vertical dome division can dramatically improve tip definition, there is concern that it may weaken the intrinsic tip support mechanism, thereby inducing tip irregularities such as pinching, alar notching, and/or a tent pole nasal tip. Moreover, this technique can damage part of the lateral support in patients with thin skin and solid cartilage; this damage can result in lateral wall collapse, alar retraction, or unequal tip uplift. In many cases, it is difficult to obtain an ideal nasal tip by using the vertical dome division procedure only. We use the modified vertical dome division technique, where the incisions are performed on both domes and a large amount of cartilage is borrowed from the caudal margin so that the lateral view of the medialized cartilage has a triangular projection shape toward the anterocaudal direction.[2] A cartilage strip that is shaped like a columellar strut is then placed between both limbs of the divided dome and is sewn together with the medialized domal portion of the lower lateral cartilages. Thereafter, a shield-shaped tip graft is placed just in front of the newly created cartilage-strut complex (**Fig. 12**, Video 2). During this procedure, the vestibular skin is preserved by undermining along the medial and lateral crura up to the dome division site. The leading edge of the shield-shaped graft is adjusted according to the desired height of the new tip. The modified vertical dome division technique is suitable for patients with thick tip skin and relatively strong

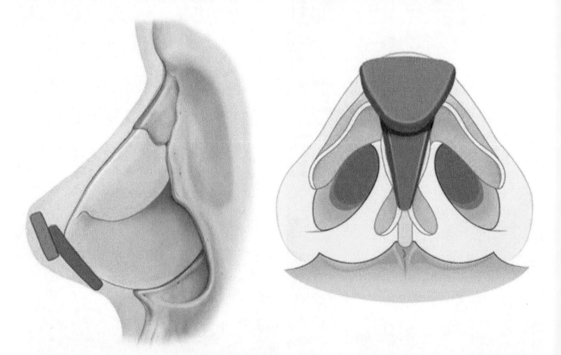

Fig. 11. Two tip graft layers. The first shield-shaped cartilage graft layer promotes tip projection, while the second layer adds further projection and a natural-looking infratip break.

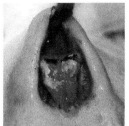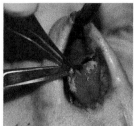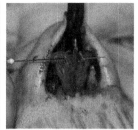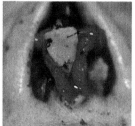

Fig. 12. The modified vertical dome division technique. The medialized domal portion of the lower lateral cartilages after dome division is sewn together with a columellar strut and a shield-shaped tip graft.

and well-developed lower lateral cartilage (**Fig. 13**). Complications of the modified vertical dome division procedure include excessive narrowing, alar lobule concavity, and asymmetry of the nasal tip.

Lateral Crural Onlay Graft

This graft is placed on the lateral crus.[4] We use this technique to correct alar concavity and irregularities of alar contour, and to prevent cephalic bending of a shield graft (**Fig. 14**). A unilateral lateral crural onlay graft can correct discrepancies between the lateral crura in terms of height. Functionally, it reinforces the lateral crura and thereby improves the collapsed nasal valve. Septal cartilage, conchal cartilage, and the curved outer layer of costal cartilage can be used. A possible complication is that the graft is too thick and shows through the skin in patients with thin skin.

Lateral Crural Strut Graft

This surgical technique involves dissection of the lateral crus off the vestibular skin and a cartilage graft is fixed to the undersurface of the lateral crus.[4] This technique can correct alar retraction, alar rim collapse, concave lateral crura, boxy nasal tip, and malpositioned lateral crura. If necessary, the lateral crus–strut graft complex can be caudally rotated and repositioned to the more caudally located soft tissue pocket at the inner aspect of the alar lobule; this maneuver is mostly performed to correct a cephalically malpositioned lateral crus.[18] Our main indication for performing lateral crural strut grafting is correction of an alar retraction that manifests as nostril asymmetry and discrepant nostril apex, and is caused by previous rhinoplasty (**Fig. 15**).

In recent times, lateral crural strut grafting increasingly involves more caudal repositioning of the lateral crus and graft complex to correct cephalic malposition of the lateral crus. This inevitably involves separation of the lateral crus from the underlying skin. In our experience, detachment of the vestibular skin from the lateral crus increases the probability of graft-related infection because it disrupts the circulation or causes a mucosal defect. These effects are particularly common in revision rhinoplasty. Thus, we recommend that this technique should be applied judiciously in the multiply revised nose. Notably, although lateral crural strut grafting is useful for correcting nostril asymmetry, it can be complicated by unexpected nostril asymmetry.

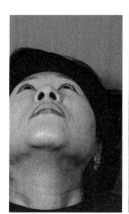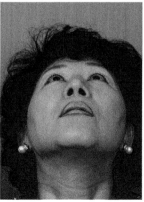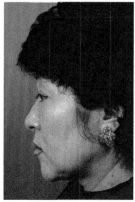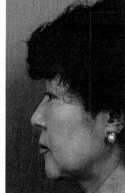

Fig. 13. A patient with improved tip projection as a result of the modified vertical dome division technique.

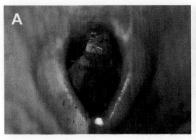
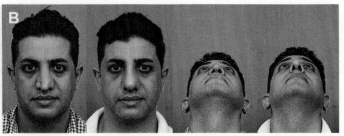

Fig. 14. (*A*) Intraoperative photograph of a lateral onlay graft. (*B*) A patient with improved right alar concavity after the placement of a lateral crural onlay graft.

Columellar Plumping Graft

A frequent anatomic feature of Asians is an acute nasolabial angle. To widen the acute columellar–labial angle, a columellar plumping graft can be placed in front of the anterior nasal spine (**Fig. 16**). To maximize the effect of this grafting, a big piece of costal cartilage can be carved and inserted. Because it is not easy to fix the inserted cartilage, it is desirable to adequately dissect a pocket that is suitable for the size of the graft. The surgery can also be performed by using crushed cartilage. Noteworthy complications are an obvious graft contour and an uncomfortable sensation in the upper lip when the lips are moved.

SELECTION OF SURGICAL MANEUVER BASED ON THE SHAPE OF THE NASAL TIP

The nasal tip shape is determined by the interplay between the cartilaginous skeleton of the tip and the overlying skin–soft tissue envelope.[19] In particular, the projection, direction, and strength of the lower lateral cartilages play critical roles in nasal tip aesthetics. In profile analysis, a tip with good definition and projection exhibits anterocaudal projection of the lower

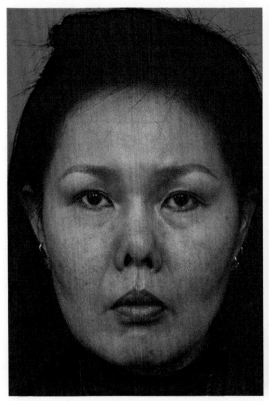
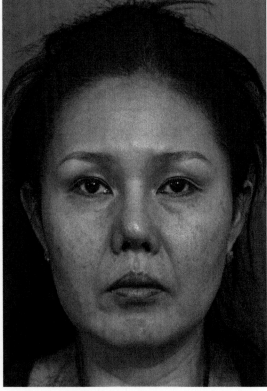

Fig. 15. A patient with improved alar retraction after lateral crural strut grafting.

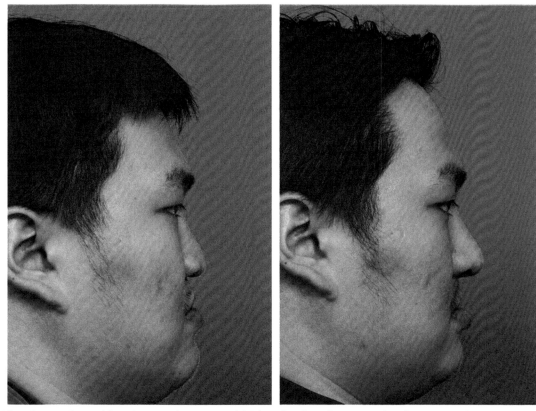

Fig. 16. A patient with an improved acute nasolabial angle after placement of a plumping graft.

lateral cartilages and slight angulation in the dome. Because patients who want tip plasty differ in terms of tip cartilage configuration and skin thickness, the tip grafting procedures that are used to meet the desired aesthetic goal must be selected and tailored based on the specific nasal anatomy of the patient.

Our analysis of the profile views of the alar cartilage of our Korean patients suggests that they can be classified into 4 different types, namely, a round contour (type I), lower lateral cartilage with 1 angulation (type II), lower lateral cartilage with 2 angulations (type III), and hypoplastic lower lateral cartilage (type IV; **Fig. 17**).

Herein, we describe the tip grafting procedures that will most likely provide an acceptable tip in patients with these different tip shapes. It should be noted that the aim of these guidelines is simply to give an idea of how to create a tip with acceptable projection and definition; these guidelines are not intended to serve as a strict roadmap for all tip surgeries. One can use 1 technique or combine different techniques to meet the tip refinement needs of the individual patient.

Type I (Round Contour)

In patients with lower lateral cartilage that has a round contour, placing just 1 shield graft can make the tip look more rotated. In addition, a single tip onlay graft cannot create the anticipated tip projection or a supratip break. Our preferred way of refining this type of tip is to place a multilayer shield graft that is, supported by a backing graft. Two or 3 layers of stacked onlay grafts and 1 shield graft can also create a desirable tip shape in type I patients.

Type II (Lower Lateral Cartilage with One Angulation)

In type II patients, 1 short shield graft can project the tip and create an infratip and a supratip break. Combining 1 tip onlay graft with 1 lobule graft can also generate an ideal tip shape.

Type III (Lower Lateral Cartilage with Two Angulations)

In type III patients, tip onlay grafting or a stacked tip onlay graft can easily generate a desirable tip shape with a double break.

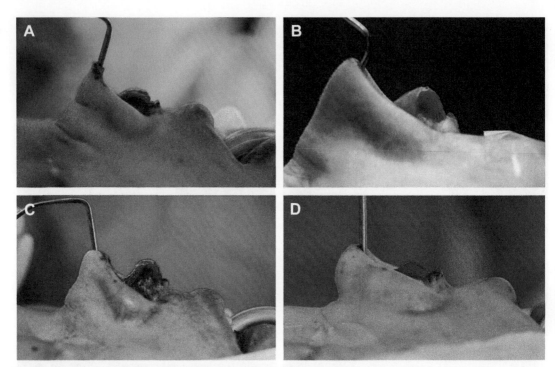

Fig. 17. Classification of the profile views of the alar cartilage contour in Asian patients. (*A*) Type I (round contour), (*B*) type II (lower lateral cartilage with 1 angulation), (*C*) type III (lower lateral cartilage with 2 angulations), and (*D*) type IV (hypoplastic lower lateral cartilage).

Type IV (Hypoplastic Lower Lateral Cartilage)

This tip anatomy usually associates with a severely underprojected tip. Its correction requires groundwork with septal extension grafts that profoundly increase tip projection and support. Thereafter, multilayer tip grafting such as that used with the type 1 alar cartilage contour may be needed.

COMPLICATIONS OF TIP GRAFTING PROCEDURES

The complications of tip grafting are not uncommon and should be carefully considered when selecting the tip refinement strategy for individual patients.

Deprojection

This is where projection obtained at an early stage of surgery devolves over time owing to absorption of the tip graft or loosening of the sutures.

Infection

This complication occurs when too many cartilage pieces are used for tip grafting, or when thick costal cartilage is used as a tip graft.[14] Moreover, incomplete closure of the marginal incision may predispose patients to infection.

Another cause may be the use of a large quantity of suture material to fix the tip grafts. Signs of infection are tip erythema and swelling, granulation tissue formation at the marginal incision site, and discharge. Tip graft infection is usually an early complication that arises within 4 weeks of the operation. When this problem arises, we remove the tip grafts via small marginal incisions and irrigate the tip area.

Graft Visibility, Migration, and Deviation

This complication often occurs when tip grafting is performed on patients with relatively thin skin, or when the grafted cartilage margin is not trimmed smoothly (**Fig. 18**).[20] It can be handled by removing the graft via a small marginal incision, gently crushing or morselizing the cartilage, and then reinserting the cartilage through the same incision.

Overprojection

This complication is characterized by a greater degree of tip projection than is desired by the patient. It occurs more frequently in patients with thin skin in whom excessively aggressive tip grafting has been performed. We usually solve this problem by partially removing or trimming down the tip grafts via marginal incisions.

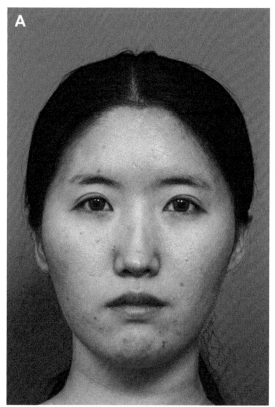
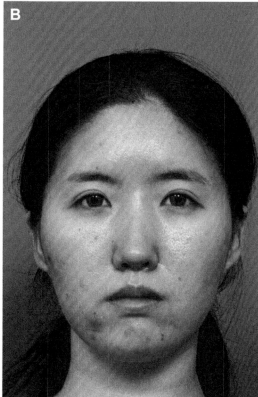

Fig. 18. (A) A patient with a visible tip graft contour 2 years after surgery. (B) The visibility of the graft in the patient improved after revision surgery.

SUPPLEMENTARY DATA

Supplementary data related to this article can be found online at https://doi.org/10.1016/j.fsc.2018.03.008.

REFERENCES

1. Rich JS, Friedman WH, Pearlman SJ. The effects of lower lateral cartilage excision on nasal tip projection. Arch Otolaryngol Head Neck Surg 1991; 117(1):56–9.
2. Yu MS, Jang YJ. Modified vertical dome division technique for rhinoplasty in Asian patients. Laryngoscope 2010;120(4):668–72.
3. Behmand RA, Ghavami A, Guyuron B. Nasal tip sutures part I: the evolution. Plast Reconstr Surg 2003; 112(4):1125–9 [discussion: 1146–9].
4. Gunter JP, Landecker A, Cochran CS. Frequently used grafts in rhinoplasty: nomenclature and analysis. Plast Reconstr Surg 2006;118(1):14e–29e.
5. Jang YJ, Yu MS. Rhinoplasty for the Asian nose. Facial Plast Surg 2010;26(2):93–101.
6. Cho GS, Kim JH, Yeo NK, et al. Nasal skin thickness measured using computed tomography and its effect on tip surgery outcomes. Otolaryngol Head Neck Surg 2011;144(4):522–7.
7. Rohrich RJ, Adams WP Jr. The boxy nasal tip: classification and management based on alar cartilage suturing techniques. Plast Reconstr Surg 2001; 107(7):1849–63 [discussion: 1864–8].
8. Gruber RP, Friedman GD. Suture algorithm for the broad or bulbous nasal tip. Plast Reconstr Surg 2002;110(7):1752–64 [discussion: 1765–8].
9. Kim JS, Khan NA, Song HM, et al. Intraoperative measurements of harvestable septal cartilage in rhinoplasty. Ann Plast Surg 2010; 65(6):519–23.
10. Kim JH, Jang YJ. Use of diced conchal cartilage with perichondrial attachment in rhinoplasty. Plast Reconstr Surg 2015;135(6):1545–53.
11. Lan MY, Park JP, Jang YJ. Donor site morbidities resulting from conchal cartilage harvesting in rhinoplasty. J Laryngol Otol 2017; 131(6):529–33.
12. Jang YJ, Yi JS. Perspectives in Asian rhinoplasty. Facial Plast Surg 2014;30(2):123–30.
13. Lan MY, Jang YJ. Revision rhinoplasty for short noses in the Asian population. JAMA Facial Plast Surg 2015;17(5):325–32.

14. Moon BJ, Lee HJ, Jang YJ. Outcomes following rhinoplasty using autologous costal cartilage. Arch Facial Plast Surg 2012;14(3):175–80.

15. Pastorek NJ, Bustillo A, Murphy MR, et al. The extended columellar strut-tip graft. Arch Facial Plast Surg 2005;7(3):176–84.

16. Jang YJ, Min JY, Lau BC. A multilayer cartilaginous tip-grafting technique for improved nasal tip refinement in Asian rhinoplasty. Otolaryngol Head Neck Surg 2011;145(2):217–22.

17. Jang YJ, Hong HR. Augmentation shield grafts. JAMA Facial Plast Surg 2015;17(4):301–2.

18. Ilhan AE, Saribas B, Caypinar B. Aesthetic and functional results of lateral crural repositioning. JAMA Facial Plast Surg 2015;17(4):286–92.

19. Daniel RK. The nasal tip: anatomy and aesthetics. Plast Reconstr Surg 1992;89(2):216–24.

20. Jang YJ, Kim DY. Treatment strategy for revision rhinoplasty in Asians. Facial Plast Surg 2016;32(6):615–9.

Hump Nose Correction in Asians

Tae-Bin Won, MD, PhD

KEYWORDS

- Rhinoplasty • Asian rhinoplasty • Nasal hump • Dorsal augmentation • Tip surgery

KEY POINTS

- Common features of the Asian hump nose are small size, low radix/low dorsum, and underprojected tip.
- Management strategy should focus on achieving ideal nasal profile and not on hump removal.
- Amount of hump resection should be tailored based on the predicted amount of dorsal augmentation and tip projection.
- Radix and tip augmentation often minimizes or obviates hump removal.
- Among various techniques for hump nose, conservative humpectomy of the bony and/or cartilaginous hump, followed by radix and/or dorsal augmentation is the most commonly used method in Asian hump noses.

 Video content accompanies this article at http://www.facialplastic.theclinics.com.

INTRODUCTION

Nasal hump surgery is frequently regarded as a reduction surgery in most Western rhinoplasty textbooks and referred to as reduction rhinoplasty. Although there are exceptions, most Asian hump noses have a small hump, and is frequently associated with a low nasal dorsum and underprojection of the nasal tip. Therefore, correcting a hump nose in Asians has distinct differences in concept and technique.[1–6]

A small hump and additional need for augmentation of the dorsum and the tip often minimizes the amount of hump removal or sometimes obviates resection itself. Hence, "profiloplasty" instead of "reduction rhinoplasty" might be a suitable word when dealing with Asian hump noses. In this article, characteristics of the Asian hump nose are addressed with emphasis on surgical techniques commonly used to obtain reliable results.

ANATOMIC CONSIDERATIONS AND CLINICAL IMPLICATIONS

The thickness of the dorsal skin varies across the nasal dorsum. It is thickest in the nasion and thinnest in the rhinion (**Fig. 1**), resulting in a slight natural convexity in the rhinion area. The clinical implications related to this anatomic feature includes the use of a curved periosteal elevator when dissecting near the area of the rhinion or hump and to avoid resecting the dorsum in line with the nasion, which results in an overresected flat dorsum.

Anatomy of the rhinion area of the osseocartilagenous vault is also another important aspect to understand when performing hump reduction. There is a broad overlap of the nasal bones above and the septum and upper lateral cartilage below. According to an anatomic study in Korean cadavers, the average amount of cephalocaudal overlap was 7.6 mm.[7] In Asians with small bony humps it is often sufficient to remove this bony

Disclosure: The author has nothing to disclose.
Department of Otorhinolaryngology–Head and Neck Surgery, Seoul National University Hospital, 101 Daehak-ro, Jonno-gu, Seoul 03080, Republic of Korea
E-mail address: binent@hanmail.net

Facial Plast Surg Clin N Am 26 (2018) 357–366
https://doi.org/10.1016/j.fsc.2018.03.009
1064-7406/18/© 2018 Elsevier Inc. All rights reserved.

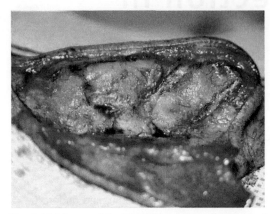

Fig. 1. Thickness of the nasal dorsal skin. Thickness of the dorsal nasal skin is thickest in the nasion and thinnest in the rhinion resulting in a slight natural convexity in the rhinion area.

hump until it reveals the underlying cartilage. In instances with bigger humps it becomes necessary to resect this underlying dorsal septal cartilage after bony humpectomy. Failure to address this issue may result in undercorrection.

There is a change in shape of the dorsal septum together with its relation with the upper lateral cartilage (ULC), as it progresses caudally from the bony junction. The sequence is from a broad "T" shape to "Y" shape to "I" shape. Resection of the dorsal septum while performing hump reduction can influence this natural anatomy. Maintaining the natural thickness of the dorsal septum prevents aesthetic and functional complications, such as inverted V deformities, overnarrowing, and nasal obstruction.

PREOPERATIVE PLANNING

The key in preoperative planning is determining the ideal profile, which is the goal of the procedure. First the level and height of the nasion is determined, which is the starting point of the nose. The variance in the starting point among different races has been emphasized.[6] Traditionally, the supratarsal crease has been considered the ideal starting point for white persons, and the midpupillary line for Asians.[2] However, contemporary Asian patients seek a higher nasal starting point. The author considers the starting point in Asians to be somewhere in between the supratarsal crease and midpupillary line accounting for individual preferences. The next step is determining the desired nasal tip posture, which is decided by taking into consideration nasal projection and rotation. The ideal profile is achieved when a line is drawn from the nasion to the desired tip. Any convexities in the nasal dorsum, such as the hump, are

resected and concavities augmented as needed (**Fig. 2**).

Other practical issues to consider include skin thickness, character of the hump, presence of deviation, and length of the nasal bones. The characteristics of the nasal hump are evaluated with careful visualization and palpation. The hump may be generalized or localized.[8] Some may only reveal its true identity intraoperatively. The generalized hump usually has a bony and cartilaginous component, whereas a localized hump is a result of a prominence of the nasal bone and/or upper lateral cartilage. A pseudohump refers to the visual phenomenon of an accentuated height of the rhinion, resembling a hump nose, which is caused by a deep radix and/or a depressed lower vault near the supratip (**Fig. 3**). Strategy in this situation is focused on restoring support and augmentation instead of resection.

We usually stress the profile when evaluating the hump nose patient. However, there are also features in the frontal view that have to be improved to achieve a satisfactory result in hump nose patients. Hump features in the frontal view include

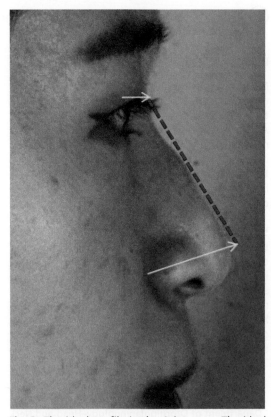

Fig. 2. The ideal profile in the Asian nose. The ideal starting point of the nose or the level of the nasion is between the supratarsal crease and midpupillary line.

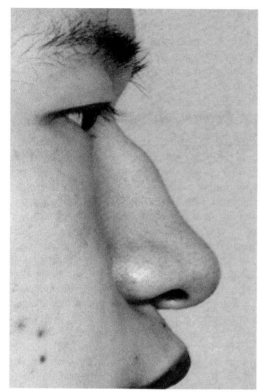

Fig. 3. Pseudohump. A dorsal convexity is seen in a patient who has a depressed lower vault near the supratip thereby resembling a hump nose.

unnatural brow tip aesthetic lines, light reflex in the area of the hump, and skin thinning with frequent hyperemia or discoloration. Obtaining a natural brow tip aesthetic line in the frontal view is as important as obtaining an ideal profile in the lateral view.

MANAGEMENT STRATEGY

Management strategy is individualized with emphasis on redistribution. The two most common

strategies used are represented in **Fig. 4**. The first is leaving the hump alone and augmenting the radix and tip, and the second is conservative humpectomy followed by dorsal and tip augmentation.

SURGICAL TECHNIQUE
The Approach: Open Versus Closed

The choice of approach, endonasal or open, is usually dictated by surgeon's preference and the need of concomitant procedures to the dorsum and tip. The author uses the endonasal approach for localized hump that does not need additional dorsal work other than augmentation (ie, spreader graft) and only needs minor tip manipulation. A unilateral or bilateral intercartilaginous incision combined with partial transfixion or hemitransfixion incision is preferred for accessing the dorsum and a separate marginal incision is used for the tip.

An open approach is preferred in cases with a generalized hump needing removal of the dorsal septal cartilage; those that have concomitant nasal deformities, such as asymmetry or deviation; and those that need major tip changes. Although these maneuvers are performed endonasally, the author prefers the open approach because it provides better visualization and comfort in applying and securing grafts, ensuring a more stable and reliable result. The only drawback of the open approach, chances of a noticeable columellar scar, is minimized by adhering to basic wound closure techniques.

Dissection and Septal Cartilage Harvest

Regardless of the approach, the soft tissue is elevated in a supraperichondrial and subperiosteal plane. The anterior septal angle is exposed, and the entire nasal dorsum visualized.

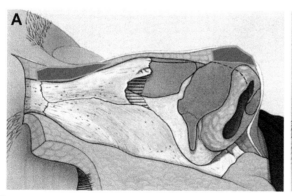
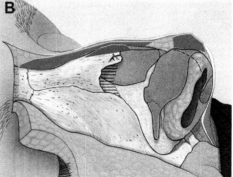

Fig. 4. Common management strategies of hump nose in Asians. (A) Leaving the hump alone and augmenting the radix and tip. (B) Conservative humpectomy followed by dorsal and tip augmentation.

When there is significant septal deviation or need for cartilage harvest, septoplasty is usually performed first leaving 10 mm of cartilage dorsally and caudally. However, when a considerable hump resection is planned, septoplasty and sepal cartilage harvest is performed after humpectomy to avoid destabilization of the rhinion.

Sequence of Surgery and Tipplasty

Before dorsal work, I usually perform tip surgery. Roughly 90% of the desired tip shape (including projection, rotation, and definition) is accomplished. The final touches are made after completing the dorsal work. The author adopts this sequence because it often minimizes or obviates dorsal reduction. It is not infrequent to find oneself in an odd situation where one needs to augment the dorsum again after dorsal reduction to match the desired height of the dorsum. Briefly, for the typical Asian patient with weak tip support, projection and rotation is usually controlled in two steps.[9] The first step is stabilization of the nasal tip. This step is the most important and key step in Asian tipplasty. The objective is to establish a firm foundation on which further grafting is added on. Stabilization of the nasal tip is achieved either by a columellar strut or a septal extension graft. Of the two, the septal extension graft is by far the more powerful tool that is used reliably in patients who have weak tip support and/or need substantial increase in tip projection. It can alter projection and control rotation simultaneously. The second step is fine sculpturing of the nasal tip. This is done by combining a variety of grafts to obtain the desired outcome (**Fig. 5**). Onlay grafts, such as cap grafts or shield grafts, are the main workhorse.

Hump Reduction in Generalized Hump Asian Noses

Many techniques for nasal hump resection have been suggested.[10–13] The author uses two types of resection methods depending on the character and size of the hump. For a large and generalized hump a component humpectomy is used. The traditional en bloc or composite resection of removing the entire osseocartilaginous hump with the ULC is rarely performed. In "component humpectomy," the components of the hump are reduced one by one, allowing precise manipulation and preservation of the nasal mucosa and upper lateral cartilage. The upper lateral cartilages are first separated from the nasal septum before hump reduction. The dorsal septum is reduced, followed by bony hump removal (**Fig. 6**). Finally, the upper lateral cartilage is trimmed separately, placed above the septum, or used as autospreader grafts or spreader flaps (**Fig. 7**). Further stabilization and reconstruction of the midvault is performed with spreader grafts. Spreader grafts are positioned preferably bilaterally in patients in whom a substantial amount of dorsal septum in the rhinion area has been resected (**Fig. 8**). The

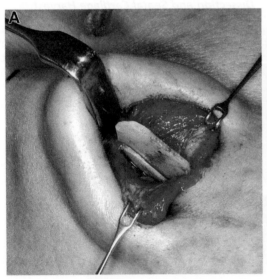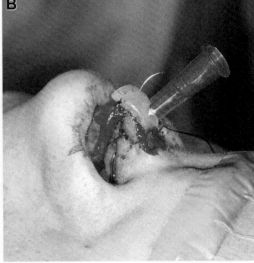

Fig. 5. Nasal tip surgery. Common steps in Asian tipplasty with a poor tip support. Tip support is restored by applying a septal extension graft (A) followed by fine sculpturing with additional onlay tip grafts (B).

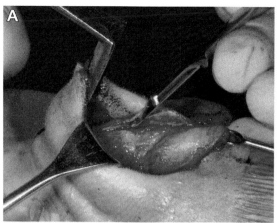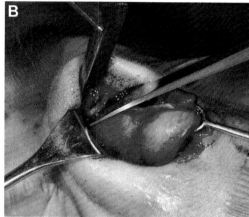

Fig. 6. Component hump reduction. (*A*) Reduction of the cartilaginous hump with a 15-blade after full visualization of the dorsum. The ULCs have been separated from the septum. (*B*) Reduction of the bony hump with a Rubin osteotome.

reasons for performing spreader grafts after a humpectomy are summarized in **Box 1**. Unfortunately, there are no studies that show the amount of cartilaginous resection and the need for spreader grafts, therefore the author encourages its use whenever in doubt.

After stabilizing the middle vault, lateral osteotomy is performed either endonasally or percutaneously in patients who have an open roof deformity, a wide dorsum, or an associated nasal deviation.

Box 1
Spreader grafts after hump reduction

- To support and reinforce the rhinion (keystone) preventing the inverted V deformity. This is especially important in patients who have short nasal bones. A short nasal bone means a short connection between the upper lateral cartilage and the nasal bone and often this connection is disrupted after hump removal causing middle vault collapse.[14]

- To control midvault width and achieve a smooth brow tip aesthetic line. The thickness of the septum increases dorsally, and excision of the thick dorsal septum can excessively narrow the midvault.

- To prevent nasal obstruction. This is the functional counterpart of a narrow midvault, which can cause nasal obstruction because of internal valve narrowing.

- To correct deviation or asymmetry of the midvault, if present.

Conservative Humpectomy in Small Asian Hump Noses

Because the hump is small in most Asian hump noses and often requires further dorsal augmentation, a simple bony rasping with minor trimming of the dorsal septal cartilage is usually sufficient to achieve the desired dorsal height or obtain the platform for further dorsal augmentation.

Using a small straight osteotome instead of a big Rubin followed by incremental rasping with small rasps or a nasal drill under direct visualization is helpful (Video 1). Bony humpectomy reveals the overlapping cartilaginous vault underneath and precise reduction of the cartilaginous vault can follow (**Fig. 9**, Video 2). The author uses the term "conservative humpectomy," and it is used in most small or isolated hump nose Asian patients. Subsequent dorsal augmentation with onlay grafts above and/or below the hump in combination with tip surgery contributes to the frequent use of conservative hump removal.

Although the overlapping upper lateral cartilage is visible underneath the nasal bones in the rhinion area, there is rarely an open roof obviating lateral osteotomies. Further dorsal augmentation can also camouflage a wide nasal base. Small amount of resection of the cartilaginous hump decreases the need for spreader grafts and rarely violates the nasal mucosa, which can reduce the risk of infection when using alloplastic implants for dorsal augmentation.

When the desired dorsal height exceeds the height of the hump there is a choice of leaving it alone and augmentation performed on top of it. The author prefers to perform hump reduction to smoothen the dorsum before augmentation. The

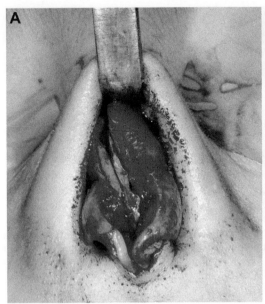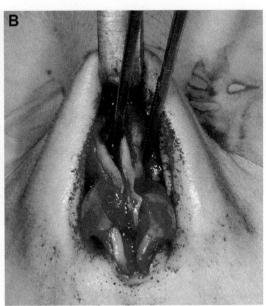

Fig. 7. (*A* and *B*) Autospreader flaps. The excess ULCs after cartilaginous hump reduction are used as autospreader flaps.

amount of resection in this situation depends on the material used for dorsal augmentation. When silicone is used, the undersurface of the rhinion area is carved away camouflaging for small residual convexity. For other grafting materials, such as cartilage, expanded polytetrafluoroethylene (ePTFE), and homologous fascia, complete humpectomy is performed because it is better to perform a uniform augmentation, which leaves less chance of an irregular dorsum and/or residual convexity.

Final Touch: Dorsal Augmentation and Tip Refinement

Dorsal augmentation is performed to achieve the ideal dorsal profile and camouflage any remaining irregularities. This is in the form of radix

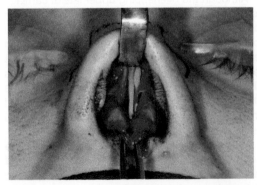

Fig. 8. Spreader grafts. A thick spreader graft placed unilaterally (*left*) on the dorsal septum.

augmentation or radix and dorsal augmentation (**Fig. 10**). The latter has the advantage of a smooth and gapless transition in thin-skinned patients. Careful palpation with wet gloves is important for detecting irregularities after humpectomy.

Final refinement of the tip is performed at the end to achieve a harmonious nose. To obtain a favorable facial balance together with a harmonious nose, it is advisable to consider genioplasty in patients who have a retruded chin.

CASE 1

A 23-year-old male patient presented with a hump nose. Analysis of his nose revealed a true, generalized hump, low radix, slightly underprojected nasal tip, combined reverse C-shaped deviation, and moderate thickness skin (**Fig. 11**). Operative techniques included the following:

- Open approach and degloving of the nose and septum including detachment of the ULC from the septum.
- Septoplasty and septal cartilage harvest. Caudal relocation to the anterior nasal spine (ANS).
- Component humpectomy: resection of the dorsal cartilaginous hump with a 15-blade incremental reduction of the bony hump with Rubin osteotome and rasp and trimming of the ULC with scissors.
- Unilateral spreader graft on the right to correct deviation and control width of dorsum.
- Tip adjustment using strut and onlay graft.

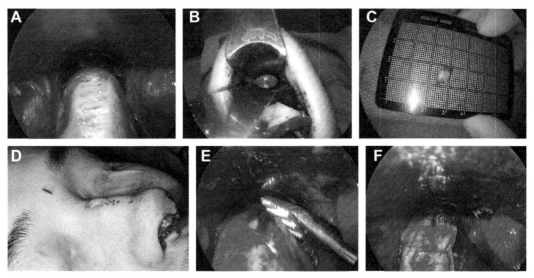

Fig. 9. Conservative humpectomy in a small Asian hump nose. (A) Visualization of the hump. (B–E) Bony humpectomy using small osteotome and rasp. (F) Bony humpectomy reveals overlapping cartilaginous vault in the rhinion that is further resected.

- Medial and lateral osteotomy to correct deviation.
- Radix augmentation with homologous fascia.
- Final tip adjustment with cap and shield graft.
- Supratip dorsal only graft with crushed cartilage.

The postoperative pictures taken 6 months after the operation show a balanced profile on lateral and oblique views, with the radix augmented and tip slightly rotated and augmented. The nose is straight on the frontal view, with smooth brow tip esthetic (BTE) lines of adequate width.

CASE 2

A 19-year-old male patient complained of a bump on his nose. Characteristics of his nose included a small hump with a low radix, slightly underprojected tip, and irregular BTE lines with moderate thickness skin (**Fig. 12**). Operative technique included the following:

- Endonasal approach. Intercartilagenous approach connected to a hemitransfixion incision to approach the dorsum.
- Septoplasty and septal cartilage harvest.

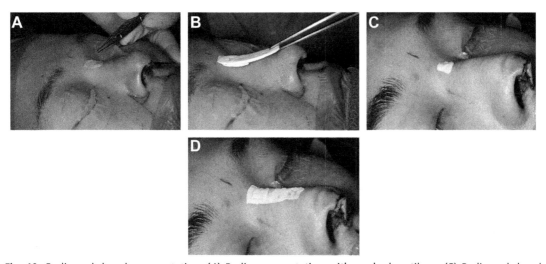

Fig. 10. Radix and dorsal augmentation. (A) Radix augmentation with crushed cartilage. (B) Radix and dorsal augmentation with e-PTFE. (C) Radix augmentation with periosteum. (D) Radix and dorsal augmentation with perichondrium.

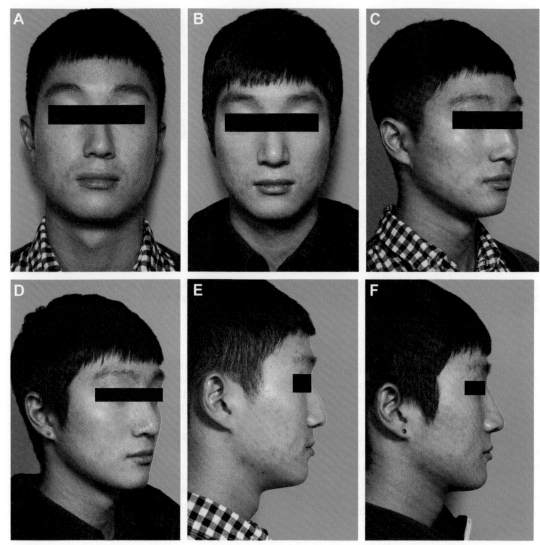

Fig. 11. Case 1. Pre (*A,C,E*) and postoperative (*B,D,F*) facial photographs of a 23 year-old male patient with a true, generalized hump, low radix, slightly underprojected nasal tip, and combined reverse C shaped deviation. A component humpectomy was performed together with radix augmentation.

- Tipplasty via bilateral marginal incisions. Columellar strut and cap graft.
- Conservative humpectomy using rasp for the bony hump and trimming of cartilaginous rhinion with a 15-blade.
- Radix augmentation with e-PTFE sheet.

Postoperative pictures 1 year after the operation show a balanced profile on lateral and oblique views and improved BTE lines in the frontal view.

COMPLICATIONS AND MANAGEMENT
Inverted "V" Deformity

Causes of an inverted V deformity are middle vault collapse, failure to close the bony open roof, and detachment of the upper lateral cartilage from the nasal bones (**Fig. 13**). Although not common in small Asian humps, patients who have short nasal bones are predisposed. Short nasal bones imply a short overlap between the cartilaginous vault and the nasal bones and this connection can be disrupted during hump removal. Techniques to prevent middle vault collapse include spreader grafts, binding sutures, and camouflage onlay grafts.

Residual Convexity

Causes of residual convexity include too conservative humpectomy, inadequate augmentation or resorption of radix implant, and tip drooping.

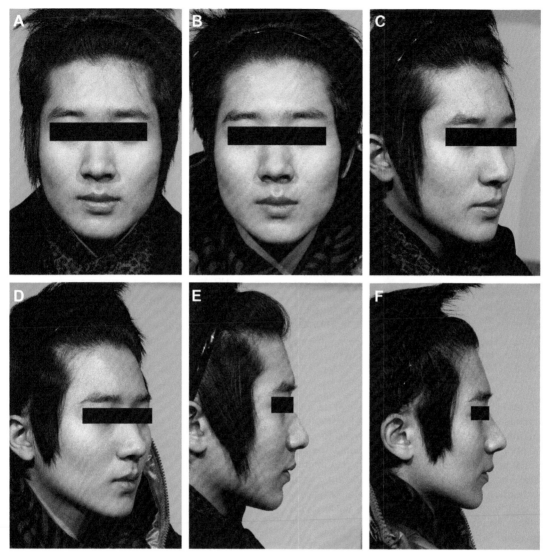

Fig. 12. Case 2. Pre (*A,C,E*) and postoperative (*B,D,F*) facial photographs of a 19 year-old male patient with a small hump with a low radix and slightly underprojected tip. A conservative humpectomy was performed together with radix and tip augmentation.

Failure in the estimation of the appropriate amount of hump removal together with failure to execute one or more steps of hump removal are some of the causes of a residual true hump.

Irregularity of the Dorsum

The dorsum, especially the rhinion where the skin is thinnest, is prone to show irregularities on long-term follow-up. Visible dorsal irregularities are a common cause for secondary rhinoplasty.[15] The thick dorsal skin of the Asian nose and simultaneous dorsal augmentation with hump removal can reduce the chances of dorsal irregularities. Verification of a smooth dorsum by careful palpation after redraping the skin is essential. Continuous augmentation of the dorsum from radix to the supratip can also reduce this problem. When performing radix augmentation, one should try to avoid using solid cartilage grafts because they are prone to show. The author prefers soft tissue grafting material, such as autologous or homologous fascia, and e-PTFE. When more augmentation is needed, crushed cartilage is inserted below the soft tissue graft.

Functional Problems (Internal Valve Collapse)

Preservation of the internal nasal valve after dorsal hump reduction is frequently emphasized in the

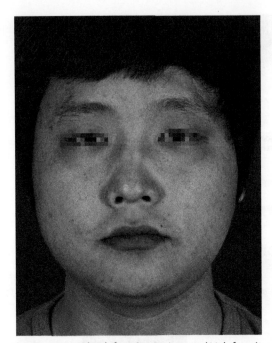

Fig. 13. Inverted V deformity. An inverted V deformity is seen in a patient who has had a previous rhinoplasty 3 years before.

Western literature. Dorsal reduction itself narrows the nasal valve. In addition, lateral osteotomy and infracture of the lateral nasal walls to close the open roof deformity can subsequently medialize the upper lateral cartilages resulting in internal valve collapse, leading to significant nasal obstruction. Techniques to preserve or reconstruct the middle vault and internal valve in the setting of hump reduction include using the classic spreader grafts, "pushdown" technique,[13] and spreader flap or autospreader flaps.[16] However, obstruction caused by internal valve collapse is rare in Asians even after medialization of the lateral walls because of the thick skin and soft tissue envelope with wide internal valve angle.[17] A previous study in Asian hump patients has shown no incidence of postoperative nasal obstruction after lateral osteotomies regardless of the use of spreader grafts.

SUMMARY

Although surgical techniques are similar, anatomic characteristics of the Asian hump nose coupled with differences in aesthetic standards dictate that it be approached in a unique way. Reduction and augmentation goes with the management strategy of the Asian hump nose, the key being redistribution to achieve the ideal profile.

SUPPLEMENTARY DATA

Supplementary data related to this article can be found online at https://doi.org/10.1016/j.fsc.2018.03.009.

REFERENCES

1. Won TB, Jin HR. Hump resection. In: Jin HR editor. Aesthetic plastic surgery of the east Asian face. New York: Thieme; 2016. p. 60–71.
2. Toriumi DM, Swartout B. Asian rhinoplasty. Facial Plast Surg Clin North Am 2007;15:293–307.
3. Jang YJ, Alfanta EM. Rhinoplasty in the Asian nose. Facial Plast Surg Clin North Am 2014;22(3):357–77.
4. Jin HR, Won TB. Nasal hump removal in Asians. Acta Otolaryngol Suppl 2007;(558):95–101.
5. Won TB, Jin HR. Nuances with the Asian tip. Facial Plast Surg 2012;28(2):187–93.
6. Jin HR, Won TB. Recent advances in Asian rhinoplasty. Auris Nasus Larynx 2011;38(2):157–64.
7. Kim CH, Jung DH, Park MN, et al. Surgical anatomy of cartilaginous structures of the Asian nose: clinical implications in rhinoplasty. Laryngoscope 2010; 120(5):914–9.
8. Jang YJ, Kim JH. Classification of convex nasal dorsum deformities in Asian patients and treatment outcomes. J Plast Reconstr Aesthet Surg 2011; 64(3):301–6.
9. Jin HR, Won TB. Nasal tip augmentation in Asians using autogenous cartilage. Otolaryngol Head Neck Surg 2009;140:526–30.
10. Ishida J, Ishida LC, Ishida LH, et al. Treatment of the nasal hump with preservation of the cartilaginous framework. Plast Reconstr Surg 1999;103(6):1729–33.
11. Rohrich RJ, Muzaffar AR, Janis JE. Component dorsal hump reduction: the importance of maintaining dorsal aesthetic lines in rhinoplasty. Plast Reconstr Surg 2004;114(5):1298–308.
12. Skoog T. A method of hump reduction in rhinoplasty: a technique for preservation of the nasal roof. Arch Otolaryngol 1966;83:283–7.
13. Hall JA, Peters MD, Hilger PA. Modification of the Skoog dorsal reduction for preservation of the middle nasal vault. Arch Facial Plast Surg 2004;6:105–10.
14. Sheen JH. Spreader graft: a method of reconstructing the roof of the middle nasal vault following rhinoplasty. Plast Reconstr Surg 1984;73:230–9.
15. Won TB, Jin HR. Revision rhinoplasty in Asians. Ann Plast Surg 2010;65(4):379.
16. Gruber RP, Park E, Newman J, et al. The spreader flap in primary rhinoplasty. Plast Reconstr Surg 2007;119(6):1903–10.
17. Suh MW, Jin HR, Kim JH. Computed tomography versus nasal endoscopy for the measurement of the internal nasal valve angle in Asians. Acta Otolaryngol 2008;128(6):675–9.

Alar Base Reduction and Alar-Columellar Relationship

Ji Yun Choi, MD, PhD

KEYWORDS

- Alar base reduction • Alar columella relationship • Alar retraction • Wide alar base

KEY POINTS

- Creating an aesthetically balanced alar base is an important supplementary surgical technique in rhinoplasty for Asian patients because many Asians have noses with a broad alar base.
- For proper assessment of the nasal base width, a clear distinction should be made between the width of the alar base and the degree of alar flare.
- Nasal sill reduction involves the complete resection of skin and underlying soft tissues at the location of the nostril sill to make the alar base narrower.
- Lateral alar reduction from the base of the alar lobule to just above the alar facial groove improves excessive alar flare but does not narrow the nostril.
- The goal is to accomplish a natural result and preserve the natural curvature of the lateral alar and function.

BACKGROUND

The alar base plays an important role in the overall appearance and balance of the nose. Despite this, it is not often evaluated independently during preoperative nasal examinations, and, thus, it often exhibits imperfections during secondary rhinoplasty. Some of these imperfections are recognized easily, whereas others are subtle and are only identified during a detailed examination by the surgeon. Some are primary deformities that were not addressed initially, whereas others develop as secondary deformities, such as excessive alar flaring, which can develop after reduction of tip projection.[1]

Many studies have indicated that between 15% and 90% of rhinoplasty procedures involve manipulation of the alar base.[2] In particular, many Asians have noses with a broad alar base, and, thus, the creation of an aesthetically balanced alar base is an important

supplementary goal of rhinoplasty performed on Asian patients.

ANATOMY

The effects of skeletal muscles on the positions of the nasal base and alar remain poorly understood. The dilator naris muscle comprises the main muscular component of the alar lobule. It originates from the lateral crus of the lower lateral cartilage and inserts directly onto the alar skin. Contraction of this muscle helps open the nostril.

The nasalis muscle is located within the nose. It works like a sphincter to compress the nasal cartilage and, therefore, is also known as the nasalis compressor. Furthermore, it depresses the tip of the nose while elevating the corners of the nostrils. This flexing and retracting within the nose is commonly referred to as nostril flaring. The muscle originates in the maxillary part of the skull and

Disclosure: The author has nothing to disclose.
Department of Otorhinolaryngology, Chosun University College of Medicine, 365 Pilmun-daero, Dong-gu, Gwangju 61452, Korea
E-mail address: happyent@naver.com

Facial Plast Surg Clin N Am 26 (2018) 367–375
https://doi.org/10.1016/j.fsc.2018.03.010
1064-7406/18/© 2018 Elsevier Inc. All rights reserved.

inserts into the nasal bone. The primary purpose of the levator labii superioris alaeque nasi is to dilate the nostrils and elevate the upper lip. It arises from the nasal process of the maxilla, passes downward and laterally, and divides into 2 parts that insert into the alar cartilage and upper lip, respectively. The depressor septi nasi constricts the nostrils. It emerges from the upper jaw's incisive fossa—a bone opening in the front-center of the roof of the mouth—and inserts into both the septum and the alar posterior side. The depressor septi is a direct antagonist of the other nasal muscles, drawing the alar of the nose downward and thereby constricting the aperture of the nostrils (**Fig. 1**).

The ala contacts the nasal side wall from above and the nasal tip from the front. As the ala extends rearwards, it becomes deeper and is surrounded by the crescentic alar groove, which extends rearwards and is generally named the alar-facial sulcus. The crescentic alar groove separates the ala from the apical triangle of the lip and cheek.

At its caudal-most point, the nose is subdivided into the vestibule and alar base. Both ethnicity and the distribution of fibrofatty areolar

tissue in the nose affect the alar base and the shape, size, and resilience of the nostrils. Inside the nasal cavity, the boundaries of the nasal vestibule are delineated laterally by the alar side walls and medially by the nasal septum. The soft tissue immediately above the medial crura of the lower lateral cartilage is called the columella.[3]

PREOPERATIVE ANALYSIS

Preoperative evaluation of the base of the nose should assess the size, shape, and symmetry of the nostrils as well as the width and length of the columella, the relationship between the columella length and lobule height, and the thickness and contour of the ala. Before deciding to narrow the nasal base, clinicians should carefully examine the caudal septum to ensure there is no deflection, deviation, or dislocation—such caudal septal deformities can lead to nasal base distortion, loss of tip projection, or unequal nostrils with asymmetric alar flare. Clinicians should then accurately assess the position and definition of the nasal tip, because alterations to the projection, rotation, or

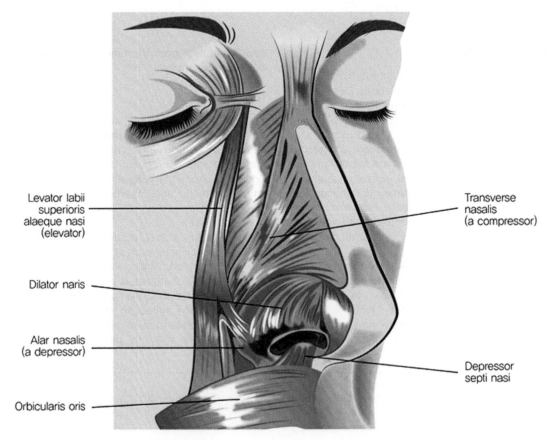

Levator labii superioris alaeque nasi (elevator)

Dilator naris

Alar nasalis (a depressor)

Orbicularis oris

Transverse nasalis (a compressor)

Depressor septi nasi

Fig. 1. The skeletal muscles of the external nose.

width of the nasal tip have a direct effect on the width of the nasal base and the amount of alar flare. Therefore, the nasal base width should only be evaluated after all required nasal tip modifications are completed (**Fig. 2**).[4]

Viewed from the base, the white nose tip—which is considered the aesthetically ideal example—has the shape of an equilateral triangle. In general, the nostrils and columella form the lower two-thirds of this triangle, whereas the infratip forms the upper one-third.[5] The lobule comprises approximately 75% of the nasal base width. Ideally, the nostrils should have a pear-shaped, elliptical, and symmetric shape. They should also have a medial incline of 30° to 45° relative to the columella's vertical axis, and they should be slightly wider than the columella.[6,7] The width of the columella should be a fifth of the nasal base distance. The general features of a patient's skin as well as the thickness of the alar side wall can be assessed on the base view of the nose. Because excessively thick side walls can negatively affect the overall structural harmony of the nose, the alar side wall should be kept at a thickness one-fifth of the nasal base's width. The width of the nasal base can be analyzed on the frontal view. It should approximate the intercanthal distance. Ideally, the width of the nasal base should comprise one-fifth of the total facial width, and it must be equal to the width of 1 eye.[3] According to Guyuron, the alar base width should be 1 mm wider than the intercanthal distance on both sides.[1] Furthermore, an alar base reduction is likely necessary when the nasal base is 2 mm wider than the intercanthal distance.[3]

Farkas and colleagues[6] reported the variation in the nostril axes of African American, Asian, and mestizo subjects. In leptorrhine noses, the ideal interalar distance is approximately equal to the intercanthal distance. In most Asian noses, however, the distance should be wider.[6] Specifically,

Sim and colleagues[8] reviewed the facial features of 100 southern Chinese women and compared them with those of white North American women. They found that southern Chinese faces more often had a nasal width greater than the intercanthal distance. In addition, the ala were more flared, and the nostrils were more horizontally oriented.[8]

To assess the nasal base width properly, clinicians must distinguish the width of the alar base from the degree of alar flare.

ALAR BASE SURGERY

Many different factors can affect the extent of alar flaring and alar base widening, including the strength and orientation of the alar cartilage, nasal tip projection, and the insertion angle of the ala into the face.

Like other parts of the nose, the nasal base partially determines the aesthetic and functional characteristics of the nose. Furthermore, the orientation of the nostrils and the shape of the nasal base both vary significantly between ethnic groups. In this regard, nasal base modification can improve nostril shape and orientation, reduce alar flaring, improve nasal base width, correct nasal hooding, improve symmetry, and create overall facial harmony. One approach to narrowing the alar base is alar base resection, whereby surgeons completely resect the skin and underlying soft tissue of the nostril sill. Alternatively, surgeons can make an excision more lateral to the insertion of the ala. Such an approach, in addition to reducing the alar base, also decreases excessive alar flaring.[6] Lateral alar reduction from the base of the alar lobule to just above the alar facial groove improves excessive alar flare without narrowing the nostril. Surgeons can, therefore, incorporate 1 or both techniques to tailor the extent of nostril or alar base reduction to the individual needs of each patient.

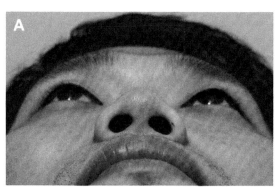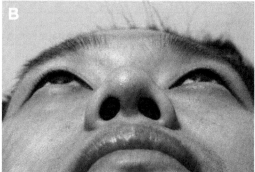

Fig. 2. These photos show the nasal tip projection without alar base surgery make the alar base narrower. (*A*) Preoperative photo from the base. (*B*) Postoperative photo from the base.

Clinicians should always consider the intercanthal distance when planning an alar base reduction. In this regard, preoperative markings and calipers are useful in ensuring a balanced excision.

Surgical Technique

To achieve symmetry with alar base reduction, surgeons must consider the type of excision as well as the amount of tissue to be removed. To ensure that the alar base modification is successful, it is of utmost importance that surgeons determine which segment of the alar base is to be reduced as well as the type and location of the excision.

In Asian patients, alar base surgery can be classified into 6 types depending on which segment of the alar base is to be reduced. Type 1 comprises long, flaring alar without wide alar base and can be corrected using lateral alar reduction. Type 2 includes wide alar bases or excessive nostril sills without flaring and can be corrected using nasal sill reduction. Type 3 is a combination of types 1 and 2. Type 4 consists of cases with a thick alar side wall and can be corrected using alar side-wall excision. Type 5 denotes any combination of types 1, 2, or 3 with type 4, and type 6 refers to cases of alar hooding. These can be corrected using vestibular skin excision (**Table 1**).

First, the position of the sill (the most inferior lateral position of the nostril) is delineated using a marker. The width of the alar base is then measured as the distance from the center to the sill, and alar symmetry is checked. Next, to confirm whether there is alar flaring, the intercanthal distance is compared with the alar width. In the sill, a reference line (the first line) is drawn by extending the line along the alar facial sulcus.

In type 1 patients, the necessary amount of resection is determined according to the degree of alar flaring, and the second line is drawn outside and parallel to the reference line. The third line is then extended backward along the alar groove at the end of the reference line. If the third line is long, the amount of resection must be increased to ensure alar volume reduction. This, however, can lead to visible scarring. A wedge-shaped mucosal resection is then performed in the nose by extending the reference line and second line inward so that they can be tapered.

In cases of type 2, the resection amount is determined according to the width of the alar base. The second line is drawn inside and parallel to the reference line and tapered toward the outer side to meet the reference line. A wedge-shaped mucosal resection is performed in the nose by extending the reference and second lines inward so they can be tapered. In type 3 cases, types 1 and 2 resections are performed together.

In type 4, the first line is drawn along the inner margin of the alar rim. After the appropriate extent of resection is determined according to the thickness of the alar side wall, the second line is drawn outside and parallel to the first line. It is tapered at the upper side to meet the first line. The third line is drawn along the alar facial groove below the first and second lines. The skin must be resected in a wedge shape. In type 5 cases, type 1, 2, or 3 resection is performed together with type 4.

In type 6, the resection amount is determined according to the degree of alar hooding, and the first line is drawn along the alar rim margin. The second line is drawn parallel to the first line on the upper side of the inner vestibular skin. It is tapered to meet the first line. The third line is drawn on the vestibular skin as an extension line of the alar facial groove below the first and second lines.

Total hemostasis must be ensured before the excision is closed. Firstly, the sill is approximated using a medial 5-0 nylon tacking suture. Suturing is then performed using 6-0 nylon to match the skin margin. To avoid step-off deformity, careful reapproximation is necessary (**Fig. 3**).

Table 1
Classifications, characteristics, and treatment of alar base deformities

Classifications	Characteristics	Treatment
Type 1	Alar flaring without wide alar base	Lateral alar reduction
Type 2	Wide alar base without alar flaring	Nasal sill reduction
Type 3	Wide alar base with alar flaring	Lateral alar reduction and nasal sill reduction
Type 4	Thick alar side wall	Alar side wall excision
Type 5	Thick alar side wall with wide alar base or/and alar flaring	Lateral alar reduction or/and lateral sill reduction and alar side wall excision together
Type 6	Alar hooding	Vestibular skin excision

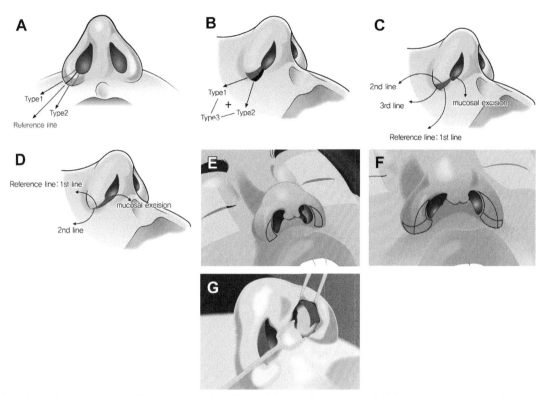

Fig. 3. Various design according to the classifications of the alar base surgery. (*A*) Basal view of type 1 and type 2. (*B*) Oblique view of type 1 and type 2. (*C*) Type 1: lateral alar reduction. (*D*) Type 2: nasal sill reduction. (*E*) Type 4: alar side wall excision. (*F*) Type 5: lateral alar reduction or/and lateral sill reduction and alar side wall excision together. (*G*) Type 6: vestibular skin excision.

Alar base surgery must always be performed conservatively. That is, beginners are often advised to resect less skin than they think necessary, because excessive resection is common. During alar base surgery, to avoid scarring, surgeons should resect less inner soft tissue or muscle from the alar rim than outer skin. Furthermore, soft tissue sutures are beneficial in cases where bunching suturing is necessary. An extremely wide nasal base may require alternative or adjunctive treatments. Base-narrowing, or bunching, sutures are placed across the length of a patient's nasal base. When these sutures are tightened, the distance between the bases decreases (**Figs. 4–6**).

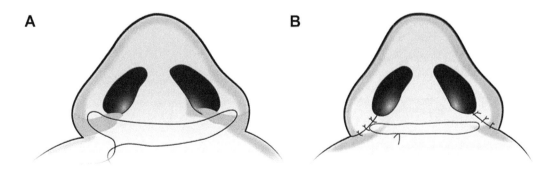

Fig. 4. Alar bunching suture are placed across the length of the nasal base. When these sutures are tightened, the distance between the bases decreases. (*A*) Preoperative. (*B*) Postoperative.

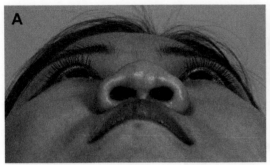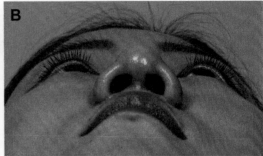

Fig. 5. (*A*) A 22-year-old female patient shows wide alar base (type 2). (*B*) Her 1-month postoperative photo shows a narrowed alar base after nasal sill reduction.

Complications

Whenever performing alar base reductions, surgeons must balance the risk of scar formation and possible alar asymmetry against the minor improvement. The following factors should be considered when designing alar base resection: flaring of the ala, the width of the nostrils, and the length of the lateral alar in relation to the nasal tip projection.

Overall, most patients are satisfied with their alar base modification. Some patients have reported a variety of complications, however, including scarring, notching, asymmetry, and overall deformity. The inability of clinicians to predict the outcome of alar base refinement is among the most concerning challenges.

In addition, alar base refinement can lead to step-off deformities, although this can be prevented through precise suturing, caliper use, and proper marking. Step-off deformities are treated using reincision and proper meticulous wound closure.[3] When modifying the alar base, it is important to ensure symmetry through careful and thorough caliper use and preoperative measurement. That said, if the patient shows preexisting nostril asymmetry, it is not possible to resolve this and to obtain perfectly symmetric nostrils (**Fig. 7**).[3]

Alar base excision provides rewarding results. Some surgeons may be concerned, however, that it can cause visible scarring or unnatural nose alignment/structure.[8–10]

ALAR-COLUMELLAR RELATIONSHIP
Background

In cases of alar rim deformities, preoperative analysis is important, because the surgical method differs depending on the state and degree of deformity, and the choice of proper procedures is difficult. Therefore, surgeons must confirm whether the alar rim is asymmetric or deformed before performing nasal surgery, and patients should be informed in advance that the deformity of the alar rim may worsen after surgery. If there is a chance the alar rim deformity will worsen, the cartilage should not be resected, and damage to the soft tissue should be avoided, as should excessive extension of the nose. Finally, the lower lateral cartilage should be strengthened and repositioned if necessary. If the alar rim deformity is already severe before surgery, clinicians must explain to the patient that the corrective procedure may be difficult, that the improvements made may be minimal, and that the outcome is hard to

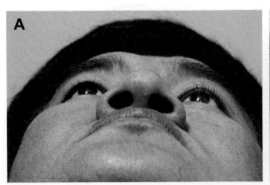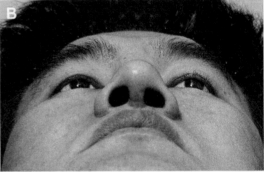

Fig. 6. (*A*) A 45-year-old male patient shows wide alar base and alar flaring (type 3). (*B*) His 1-month postoperative photo shows a narrowed alar base after lateral alar reduction combined with nasal sill reduction.

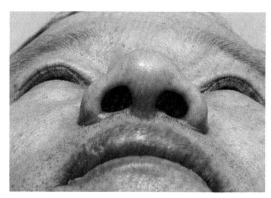

Fig. 7. Photograph shows obvious scarring that parallels the alar crease as a result of lateral alar reduction placed above the natural crease (type 1).

predict. Correction of alar rim deformities can reduce nasal congestion caused by weakening of the external nasal valve as well as improve nasal aesthetics.

Furthermore, it is essential that clinicians understand the alar-columellar relationship to ensure proper management of alar deformities. In this regard, Gunter and colleagues[11] defined the ideal distance from the long axis of the nostril to either the alar rim or the columella as 1 mm to 2 mm. Increases or decreases in this distance indicate deformity—either retraction or overhanging of both variables. If the distance is longer, the result is a retracted or notched ala; if the distance is shorter, the deformity is a hanging ala **(Fig. 8)**.[11]

Treatment of Alar Retraction

Excessive resection of the cephalic border of the lateral crus may be a common complication of white rhinoplasties. In Asians, however, scar contracture is a common cause of alar retraction, as are frequent insertion of implants and lack of adequate soft tissue for cutting.[12]

In minimal to mild alar retractions, the alar skin and soft tissue retain elastic properties. In contrast, severely retracted alar tissue represents terminal-stage scar contracture. Severely retracted ala can only be treated by addressing the altered skin and soft tissue as well as the underlying nasal architecture.

Various techniques have been introduced to correct alar retraction or the magnitude of retraction. To treat minimal to mild alar retraction, more conservative approaches—such as scar contracture release, alar rim grafts, and composite grafts—are recommended and have proved effective.[13,14] To treat moderate

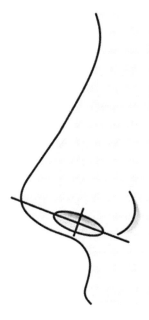

Fig. 8. The normal alar-columellar relationship. (*From* Gunter JP, Rohrich RJ, Friedman RM. Classification and correction of alar-columellar discrepancies in rhinoplasty. Plast Reconstr Surg 1996;97:643–8; with permission.)

alar retraction, lateral crural strut grafts, interpositional grafts, and intercartilaginous grafts are useful.[15–17] Traditionally, treatment of a severely retracted alar uses a multistage approach that combines several surgical techniques, such as adjacent tissue transfers, cartilage grafts, and skin grafts. To treat medially located severe alar retraction, an alar rotation flap is the most effective method **(Fig. 9)**.[12] In cases of severe alar retraction, advanced island pedicle flap provides an effective alternative. This flap confers ease of design, 1-stage operation, ideal tissue match, and excellent vascular supply **(Fig. 10)**.[18]

Treatment of Hanging Ala

Surgeons can easily correct hanging ala by removing an elliptical portion of the alar lining along with a proportionate amount of subcutaneous tissue while leaving the skin intact. The area removed should be slightly wider than the required area, although it is better to abstain from removing portions of more than 3 mm, because the shape is not attractive after over-resection. McKinney and Stalnecker[19] suggested that in thin-skinned individuals, the ala can be elevated by direct resection of the caudal aspect of the lateral crus, without trimming the lining.

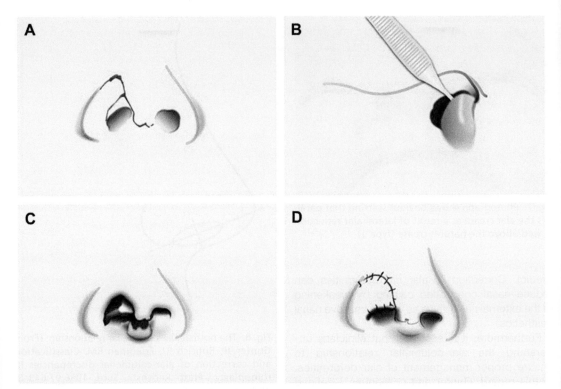

Fig. 9. The alar rotation flap. Creation of alar rotation flap and rotation of the flap and closing the flap. (*A*) Design, (*B*) Flap elevation, (*C*) Structural graft, and (*D*) Closure. (*Adapted from* Jung DH, Kawk ES, Kim HS. Correction of severe alar retraction with use of a cutaneous alar rotation flap. Plast Reconstr Surg 2009;123:1088–95; with permission.)

SUMMARY

Alar base surgery can be used to narrow the nasal base, decrease nostril size, reduce wide or broad sills, or decrease alar flaring. The authors' goal is to accomplish a natural result and preserve the natural curvature of the lateral alar and function. Regardless of the type of modification, a conservative approach to alar base refinement is

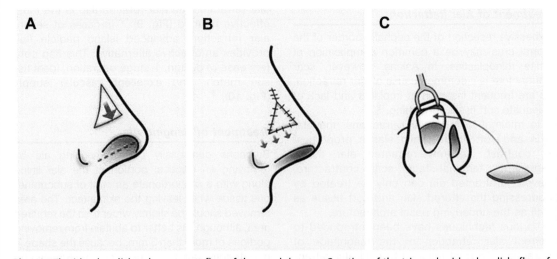

Fig. 10. The island pedicle advancement flap of the nasal dorsum. Creation of the triangular island pedicle flap of the nasal dorsum and closing in a V-Y fashion and introduction of a composite auricular graft internally. (*A*) Creation of the triangular island pedicle flap. (*B*) Closing in a V-Y fashion. (*C*) Composite auricular graft internally. (*Adapted from* Choi JY, Javidnia H, Sykes JM. New techniques for correction of severe alar retraction using an island pedicled advancement flap of the nasal dorsum. J Plast Reconstr Aesthet Surg 2013;66:1803–4; with permission.)

essential. Conservative alar base surgery is useful in cases of excess alar flare; it decreases the size of the nostril and converts horizontal nostril axes to more vertical ones. To correct alar rim deformities, it is essential that surgeons carefully examine and consider the condition of the skin. If clinicians understand ala and the surrounding tissue, support the lower lateral cartilage, and select the proper technique, they should achieve functionally and aesthetically desirable results.

ACKNOWLEDGMENTS

This study was supported by grants from the Clinical Medicine Research Institute at Chosun University Hospital, 2016.

REFERENCES

1. Guyuron B, Behmand RA. Alar base abnormalities. Classification and correction. Clin Plast Surg 1996; 23(2):263–70.
2. Willis AE 2nd, Costa LE 2nd. Surgical management of the alar base. Atlas Oral Maxillofac Surg Clin North Am 1995;3(2):65–77.
3. Bloom JD, Constantinides M. Alar base modification. In: Becker DG, Palma P, editors. Rhinoplasty Archive. 2011.
4. Kridel RW, Castellano RD. A simplified approach to alar base reduction: a review of 124 patients over 20 years. Arch Facial Plast Surg 2005;7(2):81–93.
5. Larrabee WF Jr. Facial analysis for rhinoplasty. Otolaryngol Clin North Am 1987;20(4):653–74.
6. Farkas LG, Hreczko TA, Deutsch CK. Objective assessment of standard nostril types-a morphometric study. Ann Plast Surg 1983;11(5):381–9.
7. Crumley RL. Aesthetics and surgery of the nasal base. Facial Plast Surg 1988;5(2):135–42.
8. Sim RS, Smith JD, Chan AS. Comparison of the aesthetic facial proportions of southern Chinese and white women. Arch Facial Plast Surg 2000;2: 113–20.
9. McKinney PW, Mossie RD, Bailey MH. Calibrated alar base excision. a 20-year experience. Aesthetic Plast Surg 1988;12:71–5.
10. Silver WE, Sajjadian A. Nasal base surgery. Otolaryngol Clin North Am 1999;32:653–68.
11. Gunter JP, Rohrich RJ, Friedman RM. Classification and correction of alar-columellar discrepancies in rhinoplasty. Plast Reconstr Surg 1996;97:643–8.
12. Jung DH, Kwak ES, Kim HS. Correction of severe alar retraction with use of a cutaneous alar rotation flap. Plast Reconstr Surg 2009;123:1088–95.
13. Guyuron B. Alar rim deformities. Plast Reconstr Surg 2001;107:856–63.
14. Tardy ME Jr, Toriumi D. Alar retraction: composite graft correction. Facial Plast Surg 1989;6:101–7.
15. Gunter JP, Friedman RM. Lateral crural strut graft: technique and clinical applications in rhinoplasty. Plast Reconstr Surg 1997;99:943–55.
16. Naficy S, Baker SR. Lengthening the short nose. Arch Otolaryngol Head Neck Surg 1998;124(7): 809–13.
17. Gruber RP, Kryger G, Chang D. The intercartilaginous graft for actual and potential alar retraction. Plast Reconstr Surg 2008;121:288e–96e.
18. Choi JY, Javidnia H, Sykes JM. New techniques for correction of severe alar retraction using an island pedicled advancement flap of the nasal dorsum. J Plast Reconstr Aesthet Surg 2013;66:1803–4.
19. McKinney P, Stalnecker ML. The hanging ala. Plast Reconstr Surg 1984;73(3):427–30.

Correction of Short Nose

Dong Hak Jung, MD, PhD*, Sang Gyun Jin, MD, Sang Min Hyun, MD, PhD

KEYWORDS

• Short nose • Asians • Rhinoplasty • Augmentation rhinoplasty

KEY POINTS

• A review of surgical correction of the short nose in Asians.

INTRODUCTION

Many Asians have a short nose that characteristically has a low dorsum and short columella, with a poorly defined nose tip. Augmentation rhinoplasty has been popularized to correct these features. In the past, simple augmentation was the surgical procedure most often used to address these issues. Simple augmentation of the dorsum and radix using an implant has been used, but this procedure results in disharmony of the nasal base, which results in a short nose with visible nostrils and a longer supratip lobule and shorter columella.[1–3] Accordingly, for Asians, it is necessary to elongate and augment the nose simultaneously to achieve successful augmentation rhinoplasty. Many studies have recognized and introduced the importance of nasal tip plasty, and currently most surgeons simultaneously perform nasal elongation and augmentation during rhinoplasty.[4,5]

The nose is defined by the length from the radix to the pronasale. An ideal nose has a length that is one-third of the entire facial length, whereas the Goode ratio indicates an ideal nose length as a ratio with respect to nasal projection, which is 5:3.[5] Conversely, the diagnostic criteria for a short nose may include noses that have a shorter length than an ideal nose, meaning that the length is less than one-third of the facial length. Instead of making a diagnosis based simply on length, however, other characteristics also should be considered. Therefore, the characteristics of a true short nose may be defined as follows: from the frontal view, an increased view of the nostrils, over-rotated cephalic tip, a long upper lip, and decreased nasal height are observed; from the profile view, a low radix, increased nasolabial angle, alar retraction, and decreased nasal bridge length are observed.[5,6]

When extending the nose length during rhinoplasty, the following factors must be considered: softness of the skin; presence of upper lateral, lower lateral, and septal cartilages; strength; availability of autologous cartilage for additional use; mucosal and skin conditions; and fibrotic change. In particular, extending the nose requires cartilage that is both long and strong enough; thus, it must be determined which cartilages are available and how they will be used preoperatively. If the nose becomes too long relative to the face, however, then a patient may appear less feminine and older in age, so the surgeon should be fully aware of how much should be extended from an aesthetics perspective and have the patient make the final decision on the matter.

The current practice of surgical correction of the short nose in Asians is reviewed.

ETIOLOGIES OF A SHORT NOSE

The etiologies of a short nose can be divided into congenital or acquired (**Box 1**). Congenital etiologies may be due to congenital deformities, such as Binder syndrome or a cleft nose, but their incidence is low. Most patients have short noses caused by other problems, such as developmental delay or anatomic defects and rhinoplasty in an effort to achieve westernized beauty ideals.

Disclosure Statement: The authors have nothing to disclose.
Shimmian Rhinoplasty Clinic, 375, Gangnam-daero, Seocho-gu, Seoul 06620, Republic of Korea
* Corresponding author.
E-mail address: rhinojdh@hotmail.com

Box 1
Etiologies of the short nose
Congenital
Binder syndrome
Congenital syphilis
Craniofacial malformations
Acquired
Traumatic
Neoplasm
Infection/inflammatory
Syphilis, leprosy, Wegener granulomatosis
Iatrogenic (postoperatively)
Contracted nose (host immune reaction, repeated surgeries, and infection)

Moreover, a short nose can be defined by subjective findings, meaning variation from a normal nose and aesthetic issues, which are not objective criteria.[6] The prevalence of a short nose may also change according to changes in generational, racial, and social trends and personal preferences. In particular, with westernization of Eastern cultures and the introduction of Western beauty standards, there is a relative increase in the number of Asians with a congenitally short nose, and, as a result, the need for proper correction of a short nose continues to increase.

Acquired etiologies of a short nose include trauma, infection, neoplasm, iatrogenic cause, and substance abuse. In particular, an increased number of augmentation rhinoplasty cases in which implants were used have led to a pathologically short nose, that is, a contracted nose, whereas other etiologies may be associated with rejection of the implant, resulting in host immune reaction, infection, and repeated surgeries. For such a foreshortened nose caused by contracture, surgical treatment is not easy due to many

problems associated with the condition, such as structural damage from injury and absence of cartilage caused by its use in several previous surgeries and the skin or mucosa being hard and not soft. Therefore, it is important to identify the etiology of the short nose and select the treatment method accordingly.

CORRECTION OF THE SHORT NOSE
Material Selection

First, selecting the right material for nose extension is essential. Using an implant on the tip of the nose is not recommended. The tip of the nose is a free-floating structure that continuously moves when chewing food, smiling, or making facial expressions. When a foreign substance, such as an implant, is used for the tip of the nose, constant friction can lead to complications, including inflammation. Therefore, it is better to use autologous tissues, such as septal, ear, or costal cartilage.

Recently, the use of Medpor (Stryker Corp, Kalamazoo, MI, USA), a porous high-density polyethylene implant, has increased for extending the tip of the nose, owing to its thin and strong properties.[7,8] This can become the cause of postoperative protrusion and infection, however, and when the implant is removed to address this issue, tissue ingrowth into the pores of the material may require removal of nearby tissues together with the implant, thereby causing unintended damages to the tissues (**Fig. 1**).[9,10]

The use of irradiated rib cartilage has also become more common. Irradiated homologous costal cartilage provides an alternative rib cartilage from a cadaveric source, which is easily carved, readily available, and provides adequate structural support without the problem of donor site morbidity.[11,12] Previous studies have reported, however, conflicting absorption and inflammation rates; thus, these issues should be fully considered when using this material.[8,11,13,14] When irradiated rib cartilage is

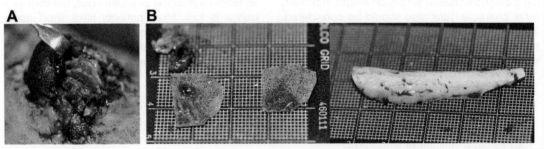

Fig. 1. (*A*) Severe inflammatory changes are shown on the cartilage and soft tissue structures. (*B*) Medpor and silicone are removed.

used only for the purpose of extending the nose, even if postoperative absorption of the material does occur, it leads to expansion of soft tissues, such as the skin or cartilage, which is not problematic.

For cases involving contracture, possible structural damage must be kept in mind. Because the material ends up being depleted and a significant amount of support is required through structural reconstruction in many cases, it is best to harvest the autologous rib cartilage ahead of time or start the surgery with preparations made to harvest the material. Additionally, it is necessary to explain the possibility of using costal cartilage to patients before surgery.

Surgical Method

To extend a short nose to an ideal length, the following steps are necessary: extend the skin; extend the support structure, including the cartilage; and extend the surrounding mucosa. These aspects need to be considered based on the preoperative decision of how much the nose would be extended. Preoperative decision also helps determine the size of the cartilage being harvested and how much of the skin and mucosa need to be extended; thus, favorable surgical outcomes may be expected because adverse events from excessive excision can be minimized.

Surgery can be divided into 2 types: correction of the congenitally short nose and correction of the foreshortened nose after surgery or trauma. In patients with just a short nose, a favorable outcome can be expected from a typical rhinoplasty. Patients with a foreshortened nose caused by previous surgery or trauma, however, often require complex and precise surgery using flaps and/or nasal septal reconstruction.

Correction of the Short Nose

For patients who have undergone primary rhinoplasty with no history of surgery, it is possible to extend the nose as much as a patient wants because the skin is soft and there is no injury to the normal structure. When extending the nose, it is advantageous to use the extranasal approach that allows precise surgery with correction of asymmetry, but the intranasal approach is feasible as well. First, septal cartilage must be harvested, but many Asians tend to have thin, weak septal cartilage; therefore, it is important to harvest the septal cartilage while maintaining an L-shaped septal cartilage, leaving 1.5 cm each in the dorsal and caudal aspects. As discussed previously, however, if not enough septal cartilage is available due to structural issues of

having a small nose, then conchal cartilage may be used with septal cartilage as supplementary material. Although extension using shield graft in the caudal portion of the medial crus is also used, the effect is not as good as expected. Shield graft that uses thick cartilage or multiple cartilages connected together apply pressure to the medial crus of the lower lateral cartilage (LLC), which may actually retract the tip of the nose in an unintended manner, such as backward pressure on the medial crus of the LLC, resulting in nasal shortening postoperatively (**Fig. 2**).

The basic concept and method for extension of a short nose involves extension of the mucosa, cartilage, and skin.

Extension of the mucosa
Because the cartilage itself cannot be extended, as the mucosa is actually extended, the cartilage is separated into the upper lateral cartilage (ULC) and LLC. When separating the cartilage, attention should be paid to the fact that perforation may occur in the mucosa between the cartilages, which may lead to postoperative infection. Performing additional cephalic resection increases the amount of available mucosa, enabling longer extension of the nose.

Extension of the cartilage
After separating the ULC and septum, the cartilage is attached to the anterior septal angle, long enough to extend the nose. This is referred to as the extended spreader graft (ESG), and it may be the most important and effective method for extending the nose. The separated ULC and septum are sutured together with the ESG. Columellar struts made with septal or conchal cartilage are grafted between both sides of the medial crus. When conchal cartilage is used, the graft has a curvature and is weaker in strength than the septal cartilage, so 2 such grafts may be needed in some patients (**Fig. 3**).

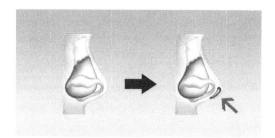

Fig. 2. A thick and/or multiple shield graft possibly induce a backward pressure on LLCs, which causes a postoperative change after lengthening of nose. (*left*) Preoperative illustration. (*right*) Postoperative change after lengthening of nose using shield graft.

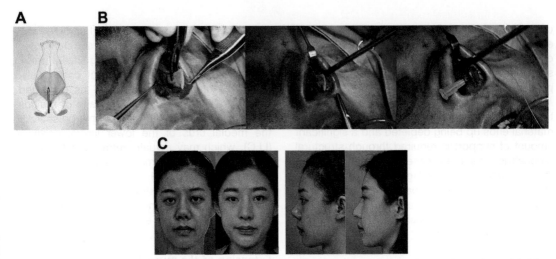

Fig. 3. (*A*) The ESG is sutured on caudal part of the septum to extend the nose during rhinoplasty. (*B*) After fixation of ESG on the caudal septum, the previously separated LLCs are repositioned for elongation of the nose. (*left*) ESG is located on one side of caudal septum to extend the nose. (*middle*) ESG was fixed firmly with septum and ULC together. (*right*) Separated LLCs are repositioned to the end of ESG. (*C*) A patient before and after elongation of a short nose using septal cartilage ESG. (*left*) Fontal view of before and after correction of short nose. (*right*) Profile view of before and after correction of short nose.

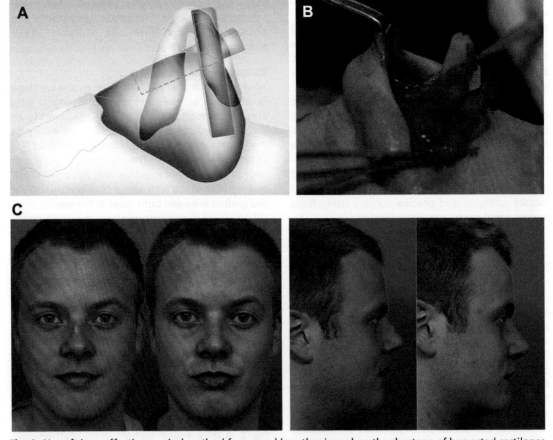

Fig. 4. X-graft is an effective surgical method for a nasal lengthening when the shortage of harvested cartilages. (*A*) A diagram shows a typical X-graft. (*B*) X-graft using a harvested septal cartilage is fixed on the caudal septum during rhinoplasty. Various types of cartilages are available to use in a same manner. (*C*) A patient before and after elongation of a short nose using septal cartilage X-graft technique. (*left*) Frontal view of before and after correction of short nose. (*right*) Profile view of before and after correction of short nose.

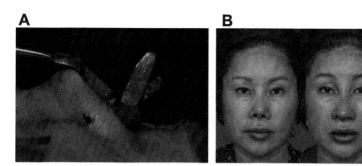
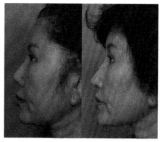

Fig. 5. (A) X-graft using a harvested costal cartilage is fixed on the caudal septum. A costal cartilage is also available to use X-graft for rhinoplasty of a deformed nose. (B) A patient before and after elongation of a deformed nose using X-graft technique. (*left*) Frontal view of before and after correction of deformed nose. (*right*) Profile view of before and after correction of deformed nose.

If not enough cartilage is available, however, use of an X-graft may be considered as well. The X-graft involves attaching 2 relatively short cartilages in an X shape on the caudal septal area to achieve extension and support, and it is often used when the cartilage is short, weak, or severely curved.[15] After fixating the ESG, a modified caudal septal extension graft is sutured onto the contralateral caudal inferior septum projecting superoanteriorly to meet the ESG in the midline, where they are sutured together (**Figs. 4** and **5**).

After connecting the supporting structure cartilage, LLC on both sides are pulled and fixed on the desired location with a thin needle, which is followed by suturing with a polydioxanone suture. Subsequently, a cap or shield graft is used for additional correction into the desired shape. Cap grafting is performed as one of the final steps in nasal tip plasty. The authors favor using conchal cartilage as cap grafts. The naturally rounded contour of the conchal cartilage is ideal for creating a natural-looking nasal tip. When using costal cartilages, it is necessary to carve the edges to create a natural-looking rounded contour. Lastly, shield grafts may be used for additional lengthening when necessary or when correcting problems of a retracted columella.

Extension of the skin

Extension of the skin is not a major problem for patients with a congenital short nose. If suturing the columellar incision site is difficult because of an insufficient amount of skin available, flap dissection may be extended up to the fontanel region, and an additional incision can be made below the transcolumellar incision using the extranasal approach to extend more skin (**Fig. 6**).

Correction of the Foreshortened Nose

Noses with severe contracture often have hard skin, not enough or no available cartilage (graft

depletion status), and injured support structures, such as the nasal septum. Therefore, it is recommended that enough discussion with patients should take place preoperatively, and the surgery should be performed after thoroughly preparing for the surgical method. For contracted noses, autologous costal cartilage is preferred.[16]

Surgery is performed after harvesting the costal cartilage first, or preparations are made ahead of time so the costal cartilage can be harvested, if necessary, after the condition of the nose is verified.

If extension of the mucosa is difficult because of fibrotic changes, then extension can be performed using a skin or composite graft after separating the ULC and LLC. If costal cartilage is harvested, the perichondrium may be used as well (**Fig. 7**).

Extension of a contracted nose requires a much stronger support structure than extension of a simple short nose, which requires sufficient strength in the ESG. If a patient cannot or wishes to not use costal cartilage and there is not enough septal or conchal cartilage, use of irradiated costal cartilage may be considered. The authors,

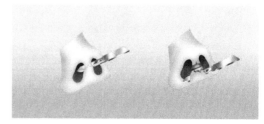

Fig. 6. An extension of medial portion of marginal incision of columella is useful to extend the nasal skin. (*left*) Insertion of blade #15. (*right*) Medial portion of marginal incision was extended below the transcolumellar incision.

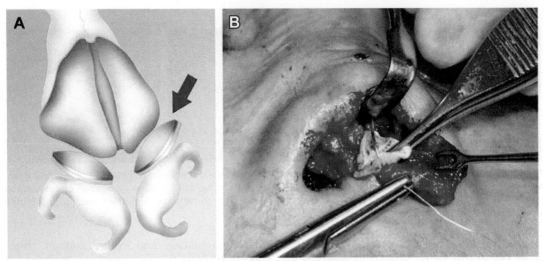

Fig. 7. (*A*) Nasal extension can be performed after separation from ULC to LLC and a composite graft is a useful graft material to stabilize between ULC and LLC. (*B*) During separation procedure, mucosal perforation can be intentionally made if severe fibrotic changes on soft tissues are observed and then it can be fixed and stabilized by the harvested perichondrium. (*Arrow*) Composite graft to cover the defect between ULC and LLC.

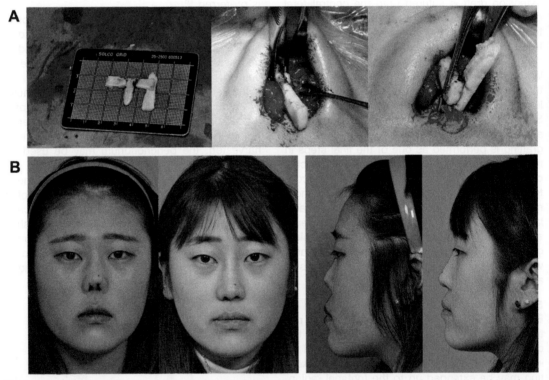

Fig. 8. (*A*) Septal reconstruction using the trussed-bridge method by costal cartilage is shown during rhinoplasty. No septum is observed due to previous surgeries and inflammatory changes. The harvested costal cartilages are manipulated to make the trussed-bridge type and fixed with columellar strut anteriorly. (*left*) Septal reconstruction using the trussed-bridge method by costal cartilage is shown during rhinoplasty. (*middle*) The harvested costal cartilages are manipulated to make the trussed-bridge type and fixed with extended spreader graft and septum. (*right*) Extended spreader graft is fixed firmly with columellar strut anteriorly. (*B*) A deformed nose patient before and after septal reconstruction using the trussed-bridge technique with costal cartilage. (*left*) Frontal view of before and after correction of deformed nose. (*right*) Profile view of before and after correction of deformed nose.

however, recommend using autologous costal cartilage for foreshortened noses. Because many patients with contracture tend to have injury to the septal cartilage, nasal septal reconstruction is necessary for a successful surgery, and autologous costal cartilage with high strength and enough availability is needed. Nasal septal reconstruction serves as the foundation for nose extension; thus, nose extension becomes difficult without nasal septal reconstruction. Nasal septal reconstruction is a method that uses costal cartilage to reconstruct the entire nasal septum as a single cartilage, and the authors prefer the trussed structure reconstruction among the various methods (**Fig. 8**).

When using costal cartilage, the authors recommend the lapping of costal cartilage (LOCK) technique (**Fig. 9**). The LOCK technique enables surgeons to maintain consistent thickness according to the shape of the ESG and strut while also providing firm support.[17] When using costal cartilage, the cartilage is usually cut into strips of more than 2 mm in thickness to reduce the likelihood of warping. Using these relatively thick grafts, surgeons frequently use the LOCK technique to fix the ESG to the columellar strut. This allows for more secure and stable fixation of the 2 cartilages to improve nasal tip projection and lengthening. In addition, the LOCK technique enables surgeons to control

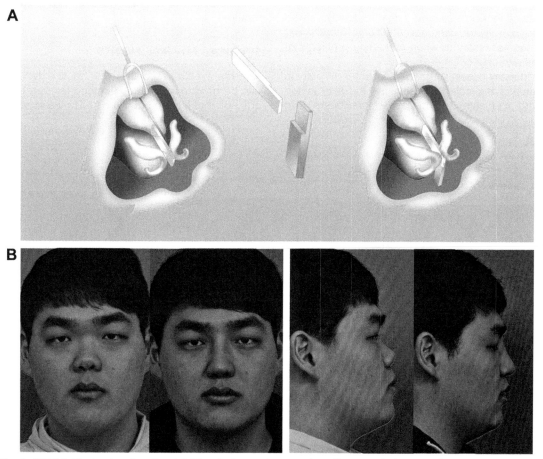

Fig. 9. (*A*) This illustration describes LOCK technique using costal cartilage. Cephalic part of ESG and columellar strut are carved to fit into each other and sutured together by polydioxanone suture. This technique allows both aesthetic and functional advancements by decreasing of columellar thickness and further stabilization postoperatively. (*left*) Extended spreader graft was fixed on one side of septum. (*middle*) Cephalic part of ESG and columellar strut are carved out to fit into each other. (*right*) ESG and strut graft was sutured together by polydioxanone suture. (*B*) A deformed nose patient before and after septal reconstruction using LOCK technique with costal cartilage. (*left*) Frontal view of before and after correction of deformed nose. (*right*) Profile view of before and after correction of deformed nose.

the thickness of the ESG and columellar strut interface. One strip is sutured to one side of the septum as a unilateral ESG. Another piece is placed in position as the columellar strut. The contact surface between the ESG and columellar strut is marked, and half the graft thickness is carved out of the ESG and then the columellar strut. These cut surfaces ensure a close fit of both grafts. Then the 2 grafts are sutured in place.[17]

Subsequently, the LLC is fixed, and additional nasal tip plasty is performed using another cap or shield graft to shape the nose. Cap grafting is performed as one of the final steps in nasal tip plasty. The authors favor using conchal cartilage as cap grafts. The naturally rounded contour of the conchal cartilage is ideal for creating a natural-looking tip. When using costal cartilages, it is necessary to carve the edges to create a natural-looking rounded contour. Lastly, shield grafts may be used for additional lengthening when necessary or when correcting problems of the retracted columella.

In many cases, surgeons encounter difficulty in suturing the columella because the skin is too hard and short. As discussed previously, skin suturing of most of the columella is possible if enough tissue is dissected up to the fontanel region and to the columellar and philtrum below the transcolumellar incision. If suturing is still difficult despite such measures, then a composite graft or subnasale flap may be useful a technique (**Fig. 10**).

Alar rotation flap can be used to correct the retracted alar, which may be present with a foreshortened nose (**Fig. 11**). The alar rotation flap requires incisions that are made along the alar grooves to preserve the arterial supply from the lateral nasal artery to the nasal tip area. Alar projection graft or composite graft can support more the alar rotation flap to manage a retracted alar. If the columellar area is injured, however, a subnasale flap may be needed (**Fig. 12**). In severe cases, reconstruction rhinoplasty with a nasolabial flap or forehead rotation flap may be required.

SURGICAL ADVERSE EVENTS

Adverse events associated with nasal extension can be divided into various categories, but they are not much different from those associated

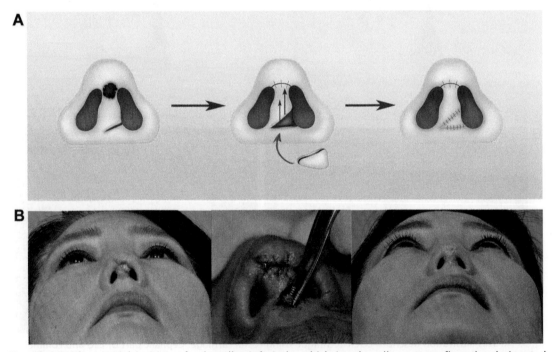

Fig. 10. (*A*) After partial incision of columellar inferiorly, which is columellar rotator flap, the designated composite graft is located inferior to columellar. (*left*) Partial incision of columellar inferiorly. (*middle*) columellar flap was rotated and sutured to cover the defect, and composite graft was located to donor site. (*right*) Composite graft was sutured to cover the defect of donor site. (*B*) A patient before and after columellar rotator flap and composite graft. (*left*) Patient before columellar rotator flap and composite graft. (*middle*) Intraoperative photograph of columellar rotator flap and composite graft. (*right*) Patient after columellar rotator flap and composite graft.

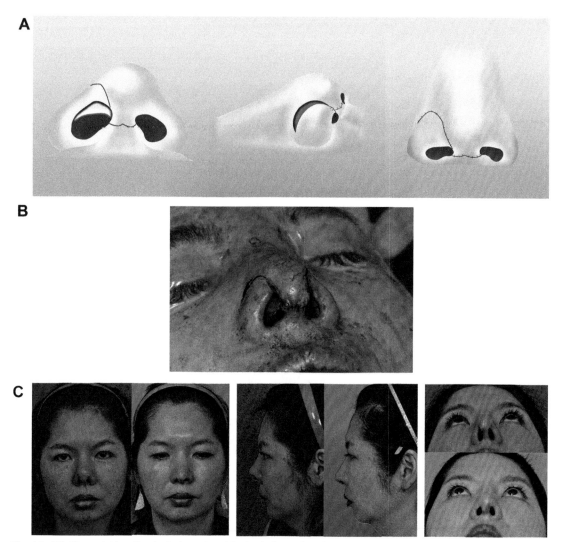

Fig. 11. (A) Alar rotation flap is designed and incised along the alar groove, which preserve an arterial supply on nasal tip area. (*left*) The design of alar rotation flap. (*middle*) Alar rotation flap was designed and incised along the alar groove, which preserve an arterial supply on nasal tip area. (*right*) The illustration after alar rotation flap. (B) Intraoperative photograph of bilateral alar rotation flap. (C) Patients before and after either unilateral or bilateral alar rotation flap management. (*left*) The frontal view before and after bilateral alar rotation flap management. (*middle*) The profile view before and after bilateral alar rotation flap management. (*right*) The basal view before and after bilateral alar rotation flap management.

with typical rhinoplasty. These can be viewed from aesthetic and surgical perspectives, where the nasal length is slightly long or short postoperatively may mean a negative aesthetic outcome despite the surgery itself being successful. Moreover, because extending the nose can sometimes result in polly beak deformity, precautions should be taken accordingly[18] (**Fig. 13**).

Adverse events that can occur from the surgery are much more broad and extensive. First, inflammation may occur, and because patients with a contracted nose may have a history of nasal inflammation, precautions are needed for preoperative and postoperative use of antibiotics.

Furthermore, because the extension applies strong force, asymmetry or bending is common. Particular attention should be paid to columellar sloping that can cause asymmetric nostrils. A scar may remain at the site of incision after using an alar rotation flap, which may require correction using Z-plasty (**Fig. 14**). When using costal cartilage, the cartilage may become

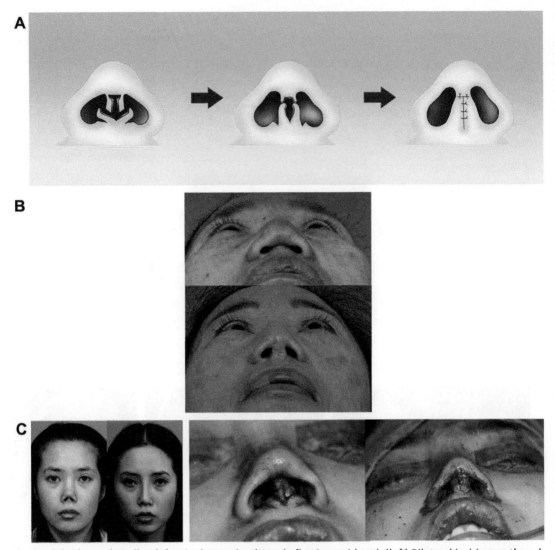

Fig. 12. (*A*) When columellar defect is observed, subnasale flap is considered. (*left*) Bilateral incision on the subnasale region. (*middle*) Remnant skin is inserted into the defect created by the subnasale flap and the most distal part is closed primarily. (*right*) The wound edges are closed using 6-0 nylon. (*B*) Basal view before and after subnasle flap. (*C*) Patients before and after subnasale flap. (*left*) Frontal view before and after subnasale flap. (*middle*) Intraoperative photograph of bilateral incision on the subnasale region. (*right*) Intraoperative photograph after subnasale flap to reconstruct columella.

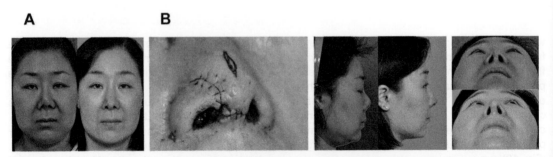

Fig. 13. To extend the nose may cause polly beak deformity that dorsal skin resection with alar rotation flap may be required to manage. (*A*) Intraoperative photograph of alar rotation flap and dorsal skin resection. (*B*) (*left*) Fontal view before and 4 weeks after dorsal skin resection and alar rotation flap. (*middle*) Profile view before and 4 weeks after dorsal skin resection and alar rotation flap. (*right*) Basal view before and 4 weeks after dorsal skin resection and alar rotation flap.

A   B

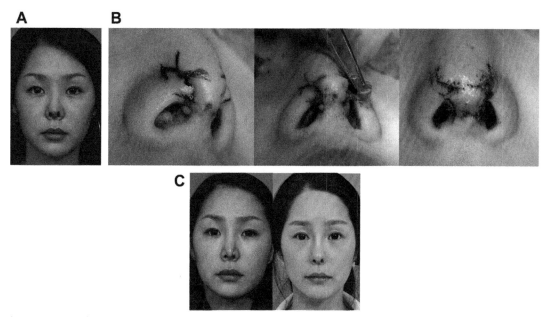

Fig. 14. A scar after alar rotation flap is managed using by a single and/or multiple Z-plasties. (*A*) Preoperative photograph with severely retracted nostril on both sides. (*B*) (left) design for double z-plasty for correction of scar after alar rotation flap. (middle) full thickness incision and dissection for double z-plasty. (*right*) intraoperative photograph after double z-plasty for correction of scar after alar rotation flap. (*C*) Frontal view before and after double z-plasty for correction of scar after alar rotation flap.

curved due to warping, and it is difficult to accurately predict and prevent such curving. When tension and hypovascularity of the nasal tip area and columellar incision site occur, skin necrosis may develop due to a poor skin condition and blood supply; therefore, great care should be taken during the surgery to ensure that excessive tension is not applied to the skin[16] (**Fig. 15**).

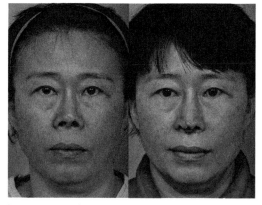

Fig. 15. Depending on skin condition and blood supply, skin necrosis on nasal tip area may occur. (left) Preoperative photograph. (*right*) Skin necrosis on the nasal tip after rhinoplasty.

SUMMARY

In augmentation rhinoplasty, which is performed most frequently in Asians, it is necessary to elongate the nose while simultaneously extending the nose as well. To extend the nose, a proper understanding of the material used and surgical method is essential. It is important to use autologous cartilage when extending the nose, and, especially in patients undergoing surgery for a foreshortened nose due to contracture, use of autologous costal cartilage is recommended. When extending the nose, the LLC and ULC are separated to extend the mucosa, and the cartilage is extended using the ESG. When necessary, the fontanel and columellar regions may be dissected for further skin extension.

Extending the nose does not automatically guarantee aesthetic beauty. It is more important to determine how much the nose should be extended based on a patient's face. The final decision on how much the nose should be extended should be made through discussions with a patient after determining the nose length from a morphologic perspective and harmony with the other facial features.

REFERENCES

1. Bergeron L, Chen PK. Asian rhinoplasty techniques. Semin Plast Surg 2009;23:16–21.

2. Kim H, Han K. Asian rhinoplasty: correction of the short nose with a septal integration graft. Semin Plast Surg 2015;29:269–77.

3. Lam SM, Kim YK. Augmentation rhinoplasty of the Asian nose with the "bird" silicone implant. Ann Plast Surg 2003;51:249–56.

4. Guyuron B, Varghai A. Lengthening the nose with a tongue-and-groove technique. Plast Reconstr Surg 2003;111:1533–9 [discussion: 1540–1].

5. Katira K, Guyuron B. Contemporary techniques for effective nasal lengthening. Facial Plast Surg Clin North Am 2015;23:81–91.

6. Ponsky DC, Harvey DJ, Khan SW, et al. Nose elongation: a review and description of the septal extension tongue-and-groove technique. Aesthet Surg J 2010;30:335–46.

7. Kim J, Kim J, Uhm KI, et al. Secondary cleft nasal deformity correction using bioabsorbable mesh. J Craniofac Surg 2016;27:1143–6.

8. Suh MK, Ahn ES, Kim HR, et al. A 2-year follow-up of irradiated homologous costal cartilage used as a septal extension graft for the correction of contracted nose in Asians. Ann Plast Surg 2013;71: 45–9.

9. Gentile P, Bottini DJ, Cervelli V. Reconstruction of the nasal dorsum with Medpor implants. J Craniofac Surg 2007;18:1506–8.

10. Peled ZM, Warren AG, Johnston P, et al. The use of alloplastic materials in rhinoplasty surgery: a meta-analysis. Plast Reconstr Surg 2008;121:85e–92e.

11. Demirkan F, Arslan E, Unal S, et al. Irradiated homologous costal cartilage: versatile grafting material for rhinoplasty. Aesthetic Plast Surg 2003;27:213–20.

12. Woo JS, Dung NP, Suh MK. A novel technique for short nose correction: hybrid septal extension graft. J Craniofac Surg 2016;27:e44–8.

13. Kridel RW, Ashoori F, Liu ES, et al. Long-term use and follow-up of irradiated homologous costal cartilage grafts in the nose. Arch Facial Plast Surg 2009; 11:378–94.

14. Lefkovits G. Irradiated homologous costal cartilage for augmentation rhinoplasty. Ann Plast Surg 1990; 25:317–27.

15. Jung DH, Loh I. The "X-graft" for nasal tip surgery. Plast Reconstr Surg 2011;128:79e–80e.

16. Jung DH, Moon HJ, Choi SH, et al. Secondary rhinoplasty of the Asian nose: correction of the contracted nose. Aesthet Plast Surg 2004;28:1–7.

17. Jung DH, Joshi A, Chang GU, et al. Lapping of costal cartilage technique: a key step in stabilizing and reducing the bulk of costal cartilage used in rhinoplasty. JAMA Facial Plast Surg 2015;17:153–5.

18. Jung DH, Lin RY, Jang HJ, et al. Correction of pollybeak and dimpling deformities of the nasal tip in the contracted, short nose by the use of a supratip transposition flap. Arch Facial Plast Surg 2009;11: 311–9.

Rhinoplasty for South East Asian Nose

Eduardo C. Yap, MD, FPSO-HNS*

KEYWORDS

- South East Asian • Rhinoplasty • Surgical approach • Sail excision • Vestibular groove
- Hanging ala

KEY POINTS

- South East Asian noses are usually small with voluminous thick skin, low dorsum, wide and hanging ala, bulbous tip, and retracted premaxilla.
- South East Asian noses possess characteristics that are different from other ethnic noses; the chronology of surgery is also different.
- In general, the following alterations are needed: dorsal augmentation, counterrotation and projection of the tip, and lastly correction of hanging ala and alar flare/base.

INTRODUCTION

South East Asia comprises a population mainly of Malay origin. The noses are usually small with voluminous thick skin, low dorsum, wide and hanging ala, bulbous tip, and retracted premaxilla (**Fig. 1**). The surgical approach of rhinoplasty for these type of noses is different from the usual. In general, the following are needed: dorsal augmentation, counterrotation and projection of the tip, and lastly correction of hanging ala and alar flare/base.

Septal and conchal cartilage are commonly used; however, costal cartilage may be used in secondary cases where septum is depleted. The scope of surgery (not necessarily in order) requires the following: (1) a strong structural framework using the central septal cartilage as septal extension graft (SEG), (2) contoured framework using conchal cartilage (eg, tip grafts), and (3) soft tissue contouring of the tip and ala.

Because the South East Asian nose possess characteristics that are different from other ethnic noses, the chronology of surgery is also different. Often times, conchal cartilage are harvested initially for contour framework grafts. Then the nose is analyzed whether a hanging ala is present

by manually derotating and projecting the tip. If there is hanging ala, it is corrected at this moment because of the need of maneuverability of the alar for marking, incision, excision, and suture closure. It is corrected via excision of a triangular tissue shaped like a sail inside the nostril. After alar rim is lifted, formal rhinoplasty commenced via open approach. The septum is dissected bilaterally and the central cartilage harvested and used as support graft mainly as SEG. Conchal grafts are used as contour grafts. Osteotomy, if indicated, is done at this point. Because volume is needed in dorsal augmentation, synthetic material, such as silicone and expanded polytetrafluoroethylene (e-PTFE; Gore Tex, W.L. Gore and Associates, Newark DE), is often used. The skin and soft tissue envelope (SSTE) is then draped and analyzed whether any additional grafts are needed. The columellar incision is closed at this time and attention is shifted again to the tip. If the tip is not showing its desired projection because of the thick skin, defatting is done. Once the effect of the new dorsum and tip are achieved, the bilateral marginal incision is closed. Attention is now focused in the ala. If the ala is still flared and wide, alarplasty is performed.

Disclosure Statement: The author has nothing to disclose.
Section of Facial Plastic Surgery, Belo Medical Group, Manila 1229, Philippines
* Suite 901, Medical Plaza Makati, Amorsolo Corner Dela Rosa Street, Legaspi Village, Makati City, Metro Manila 1229, Philippines.
E-mail address: edcyap88@gmail.com

Facial Plast Surg Clin N Am 26 (2018) 389–402
https://doi.org/10.1016/j.fsc.2018.03.012
1064-7406/18/© 2018 Elsevier Inc. All rights reserved.

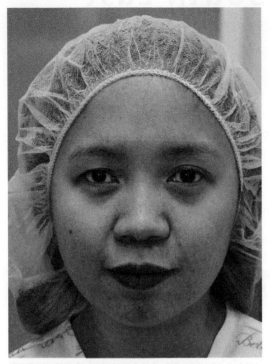

Fig. 1. A typical South East Asian nose.

SURGICAL TECHNIQUES IN DETAIL
Harvest of Conchal Cartilage: Mainly for Contour Graft and Backup Graft for Septal Extension Graft Support

Because of the small nasal structure of South East Asian nose, the septal cartilage harvested is often just enough for use as support graft so almost always the conchal cartilage is harvested for use as contour graft (eg, tip grafts).[1] Conchal cartilage is sometimes used as support for a weak or small SEG.[2]

The conchal cartilage is harvested as one piece to include cymba and cavum concha. Both sides should include its perichondrium to maintain its strength. Helix and antihelix should be preserved at all times. Approach to the harvest is done anteriorly at the inferocaudal portion of the cavum conchal bowl. If bigger cartilage material is needed, approach should be posterior for more exposure. It is best to retain 5 mm of helical crux and to use bolster dressing to preserve the conchal bow and avoid collapse of the ear.[3] Keloid can occur in posterior incision; therefore, if the patient has a keloid scar elsewhere, avoid posterior incision.

Once cartilage is harvested, it is soaked in normal saline solution. Closure of incision is done using nylon 5-0 simple interrupted. A bolster dressing is applied over the conchal bowl to prevent hematoma formation.

Sail Excision for Correction of Hanging Ala (Part of Soft Tissue Contouring): For That Extra Aesthetic Advantage in Ala-Columellar Relationship

Achieving a good ala to columellar relationship brings harmony to the tip and to the whole nose. On front view the ala-columella should simulate a gull's wing in flight wherein the alar rim is superiorly directed (**Fig. 2**). On lateral view the highest arc of

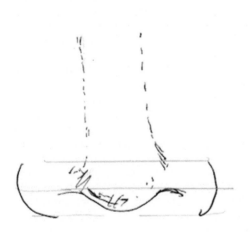

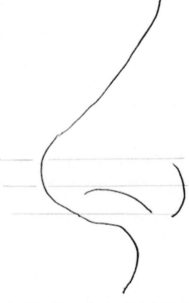

Fig. 2. The highest point in the alar rim transects equally the tip and subtip. (*From* Gunter JP, Rohrich RJ, Friedman RM. Classification and correction of alar-columellar discrepancies in rhinoplasty. Plast Reconstr Surg 1996;97:643–8; with permission.)

the alar rim should transect equally the imaginary line of the tip and subtip. There should be about 1 to 2 mm of columellar show. Many South East Asian noses have a certain degree of hanging ala. In the Gunter classification of ala and columellar, South East Asians have the class 4 to 6 Gunter classification of ala-columellar relation (**Fig. 3**).[4]

Most rhinoplastic surgeons do the hanging ala correction at the last part of the surgery. Most do the external approach, which is easy but depends on skill and experience (**Fig. 4**).[5] Usually it ends up undercorrected or overcorrected with suture scars along the thinned-out rim (**Fig. 5**). An internal approach via sail excision is the preferred approach but it needs full maneuverability of the ala and columellar for planning, marking, and surgery, hence it is done as the initial procedure (**Fig. 6**).[6,7]

There are instances wherein there is an inherent minimal hanging ala that is not grossly visible because of the upturned tip. This is elicited by manual pulling of the tip to counterrotate and project to simulate the new tip (**Fig. 7**).

Hanging ala is lifted via several methods, usually as external or internal approach. External excision is done by excising a full-thickness alar rim and then closed primarily. This method results in thinning, scarring, and exposure of hairs at the alar rims; it has no landmarks to follow so it is highly depended on the surgeon's skill and experience.[5]

The internal approach is more precise because it has landmarks to follow. It involves excising a piece of triangle that is shaped like a sail. Just like any triangle, it has an apex, two sides, and a base. The apex of the triangle is the peak of the alar rim on front view (**Fig. 8**). The apex is

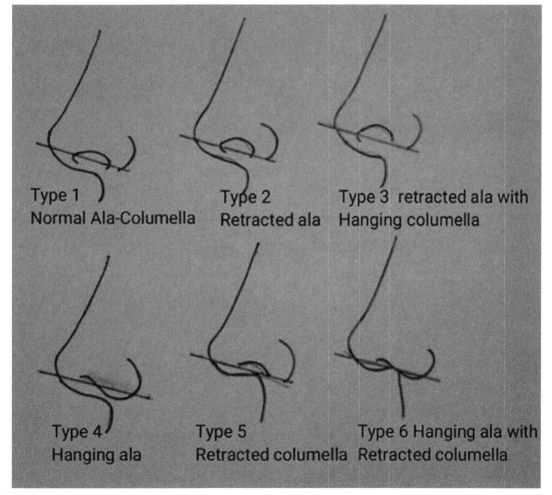

Type 1 Normal Ala-Columella

Type 2 Retracted ala

Type 3 retracted ala with Hanging columella

Type 4 Hanging ala

Type 5 Retracted columella

Type 6 Hanging ala with Retracted columella

Fig. 3. In the Gunter classification of ala and columellar, South East Asians have the class 4 to 6 Gunter classification of ala-columellar relation. (*From* Gunter JP, Rohrich RJ, Friedman RM. Classification and correction of alar-columellar discrepancies in rhinoplasty. Plast Reconstr Surg 1996;97:643–8; with permission.)

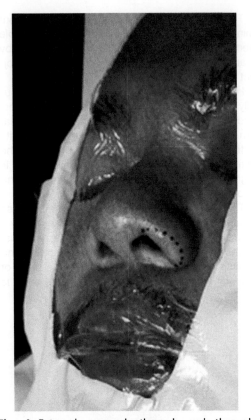

Fig. 4. External approach through and through wedge excision of hanging ala for alar lift. Suture closure is at the rim resulting to scars.

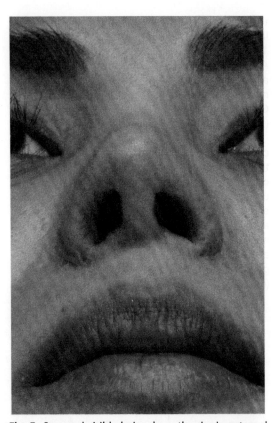

Fig. 5. Scar and visible hairs along the rim in external approach alar lift surgery.

elicited by pinching the ala against the columellar (**Fig. 9**). The caudal side is the medial alar rim. The cephalic side is a vestibular groove marked by a depression delineated by thin hair and thick hair. The depression is caused by two different planes of nasalis muscle orientation (**Fig. 10**). The vestibular groove is a constant landmark to follow; it is deeply located in hanging ala and superficially located in normal ala. The base is a line connecting the inferior end of the two sides. The base should be located 1 to 1.5 mm above the nasal sill. After identifying the landmarks of the sail, incision is made using blade 15. The skin, muscle, and subcutaneous fats are excised. No undermining is required. The defect is closed by turn-in flap from the rim (**Fig. 11**). Closing the defect starts at both ends of the caudal side, hence the caudal side coaptates with cephalic side including the base resulting in an arc shape of the new rim.[7] Nylon or absorbable polyglactin (Vicryl™) 6-0 continuous or simple interrupted are used here.

There are some instances wherein the alar rim base is lower than the columellar base (type 5

and 6 Gunter classification) (**Fig. 12**). The alar lift procedure involves an extended sail design wherein a small triangle is designed to extend posteriorly into nasal vestibule (**Fig. 13**). The maximal lift is at the area of the alar rim base.[2]

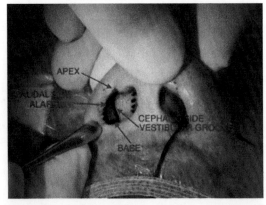

Fig. 6. Sail design. Internal approach to correction of hanging ala. A full-thickness excision of vestibular skin together with muscles and fats and then the rim skin is rolled inward and primary closure applied.

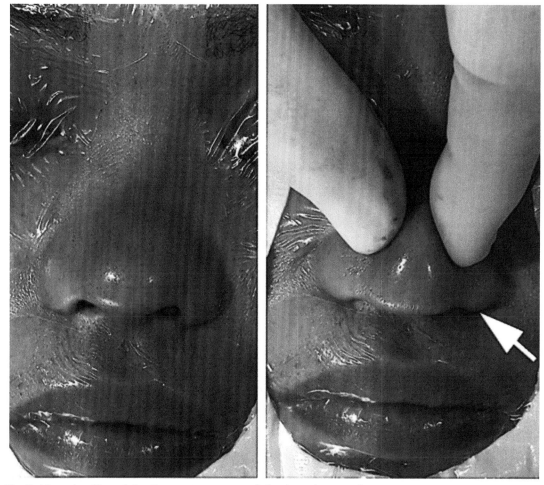

Fig. 7. Manual pulling of the tip counterrotates and simulates the new tip.

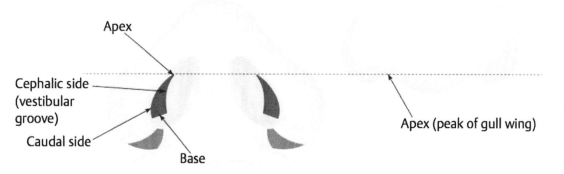

Fig. 8. Manual maneuver of pulling the tip to simulate a counterrotated and projected tip elicits an inherent hanging ala. (*From* Yap EC. Aesthetic rhinoplasty for Southeast Asians. In: Jin HR, editor. Aesthetic plastic surgery of the east Asian face. New York: Thieme; 2016. p. 110; with permission.)

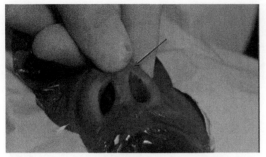

Fig. 9. The apex of the triangle in sail excision is determined by pressing the ala against the columella.

Structural Framework: For Tip Support

South East Asian noses have small and weak lower cartilage (LC). A support system has to be done for proper tip projection. Often times open approach is preferred because of the need to visualize all anatomic deformities to achieve symmetry in the framework. A bilateral marginal incision is made using blade 15 and the midcolumellar skin is cut following an inverted "V" pattern. The midcolumellar cut is usually made a bit lower and located just above the footplate so as to have more skin coverage when the SSTE is redraped over the new counterrotated and projected tip.

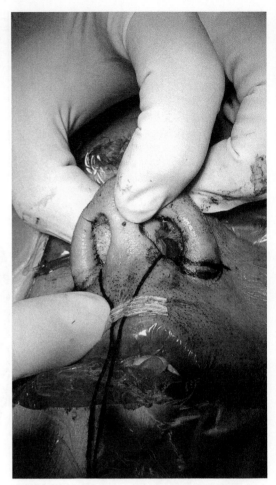

Fig. 11. The defect is closed by turn-in flap from the rim.

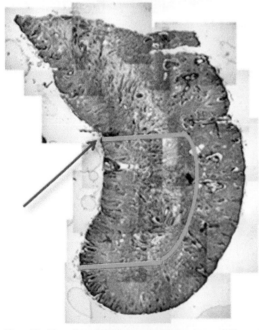

Fig. 10. The depression is caused by two different planes of nasalis muscle orientation. The *arrow* is the Vestibular Groove.

Dissection is carried out in a plane above the perichondrium in the LC and upper cartilage (UC) and below the periosteum in the nasal bone. The membranous septum is opened exposing the caudal septum. At this point, it is essential that two structures are fully mobile: the SSTE and LC.

The septum is then dissected bilaterally in the subperichondrial and subperiosteal plane exposing the whole septum. The central part of the quadrangular cartilage is harvested leaving 8 to 10 mm dorsal and caudal strut. Bony spurs are removed. A piece of bony septum may be harvested for use as support graft. The UC is usually preserved; however, it is cut away from the dorsal septum for spreader graft if there is pathology noted (eg, deviation, internal valve collapse). Any deviation noted in the dorsal and caudal strut should be corrected via suture technique or re-enforced with supportive grafts.

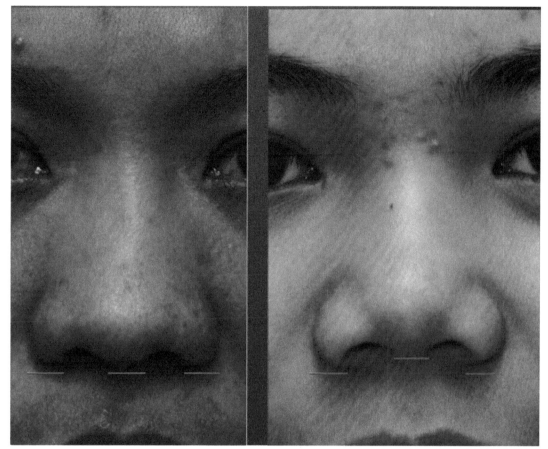

Fig. 12. Alar rim base is lower than the columellar base. Usually this deformity is in the type 5 and 6 of Gunter classification of ala-columella.

SEG is the main support graft used for tip projection and counterrotation.[8,9] There is no definitive dimension or design of the SEG; however, it is best that it is attached firmly at the junction of dorsal and caudal strut, above the anterior angle according to the vector of the new tip position. The UC attachment to the septum may be split for 2 mm to accommodate the SEG. Three to four PDS 5-0 sutures are used to fix the SEG to the strut. A vomer bone or a septal cartilage may be used as extended spreader and support graft for SEG especially when deviated (**Fig. 14**).

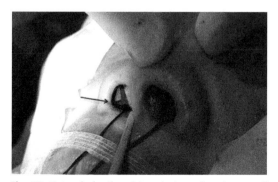

Fig. 13. Extended sail excision design wherein a small triangle is marked extending posteriorly in the nasal vestibule. It is essentially elliptical in shape with its widest defect at the alar rim base, hence maximal lift is achieved. Avoid cutting through the nasal sill.

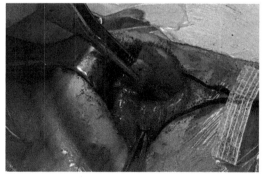

Fig. 14. Vomer bone as extended spreader graft to keep the SEG in midline.

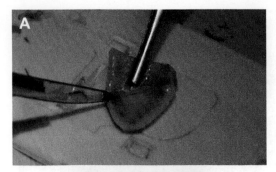

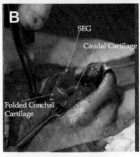

Fig. 15. (A) Midline scoring of the cavum concha and folded. (B) Folded conchal cartilage placed between caudal strut and SEG.

There are times when the harvested septum is small and weak. Folded conchal cartilage is used as support for SEG. If the SEG has enough length but is weak, a folded conchal cartilage is placed below juxtaposed between the SEG and caudal strut (Fig. 15).[2] If the SEG is short in length but firm in its attachment to caudal strut, a folded conchal cartilage is fixed at the caudal-anterior end of SEG (Fig. 16). Occasionally a long folded conchal cartilage is used as mortise

and tenon joint (Fig. 17). The conchal cartilage should be fixed at two points, anteriorly at the caudal edge of SEG and posteriorly at the caudal strut.

Once the SEG is stable, the dome of LC is fixed to the anterior end taking care that not much tension occurred while pulling the LC to its new tip position. Avoid buckling of the SEG or deviation of the tip. Fixation is done using PDS 5-0 sutures. If the lower lateral cartilage still shows convexity, cephalic trimming is done making sure to leave 5 to 8 mm of lower lateral cartilage. Attention is given to internal and external valve at all times to make certain they are patent and no constriction or collapse is noted. The mucosa of the septum is coaptated using absorbable 4-0 or 5-0.

Medial and lateral osteotomy is done at this time; however, it is best to decide osteotomy when the nose is fitted with a dorsal implant. Sometimes osteotomy is not needed anymore when a dorsal implant is properly carved.

Contour Framework: For the Shape

Contouring the nasal framework requires first designing the shape of the tip and then redefining the dorsum to fit the new tip. The grafts used here are usually conchal cartilage. The SSTE has to be redraped often to check its aesthetic improvement. Because South East Asian noses are often short and upturned, attention is focused initially in building a tip and subtip (eg, shield and backstop grafts). Once the proper length or counterrotation is achieved, onlay tip grafts are used for projection.[10]

A

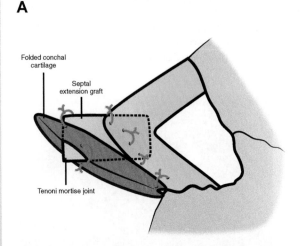

B

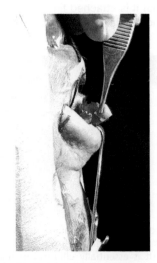

Fig. 16. (A) A conchal cartilage is folded and attached at the caudal end of SEG. (B) A folded conchal cartilage at the caudal end of SEG.

A

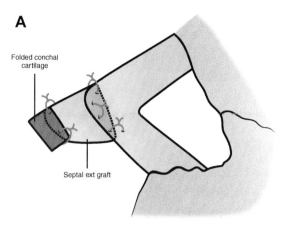

B

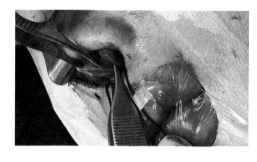

Fig. 17. (*A*) A long folded cymba and cavum concha is used to support a small SEG for projection and counter-rotation similar to mortise and tenon joint. (*B*) Mortise-tenon joint of conchal cartilage with SEG.

Once the tip is reconstructed in its desired position a dorsal graft is designed to fit the new tip. Synthetic materials, such as silicon and e-PTFE, are commonly used as dorsal augmentation material because of the volume needed. Silicon implant heals by encapsulation and the whole implant may be mobile; it is noted to calcify, contract, and extrude with time. However, e-PTFE heals by adhesion and tissue integration and gives a more natural look. Both silicon and Goretex have the occasional complication of infection.[11]

e-PTFE comes in sheets and preform. The sheets are stacked, whereas the preform has to be carved to fit well the dorsal contour. Generally, noses with shallow radix need thin sheet implant and noses with deep radix need thicker preform implant. Proper length and width is important so as to make a smooth transition of implant to soft tissue.

The undersurface of the implant should be well carved to follow the dorsal contour, notably the area of the rhinion (**Fig. 18**). Empty spaces below the implant especially at the area of UC should be filled with cartilage (**Fig. 19**).[2]

Avoid using e-PTFE sheets as filler because they may erode the mucosal lining between UC and LC.

The caudal end of the implant should be fixed to the dome so that when the tip droops in time, the whole structure including the implant droops as a unit thus avoiding the caudal implant visibility because of its detachment from the tip (**Fig. 20**).[2]

After the dorsal and tip grafts are put in place, the SSTE is redraped and the dorsum is palpated whether all desired aesthetic landmarks are achieved. Avoid a palpable tip graft because it may become visible in time. Using a rectangular tip graft to achieve a bidomal tip is pleasant looking because of the cushion of the thick SSTE (**Fig. 21**). In noses with thin SSTE a last piece of crushed conchal cartilage is placed for a better smooth-looking tip (**Fig. 22**).

The columellar incision is closed using absorbable and nylon 6-0. Sometimes a piece of 1.5 mm × 10 mm conchal cartilage is inserted as columellar contour graft and this also results in a columellar show.

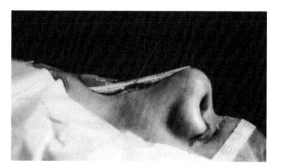

Fig. 18. The implant should fit well the dorsal surface of the nose. The area of the rhinion should be carved out to allow maximal contact of implant to the underlying bone and cartilage.

SOFT TISSUE CONTOURING
Defating the Tip: For Added Tip Definition

After columellar incision is closed, attention is made at the tip whether all aesthetic landmarks are achieved. If the tip is still bulbous, the fats surrounding the supratip are trimmed using a sinus Tru-Cut (Karl Storz, CA, USA) forceps inserted through the bilateral marginal incision (**Fig. 23**). Be careful not to trim the fat at the area of the tip. The protective mechanism provided by the overlying fats to tip cartilages adds smoothness of the tip and protects the tip skin from cartilage visibility in the future.

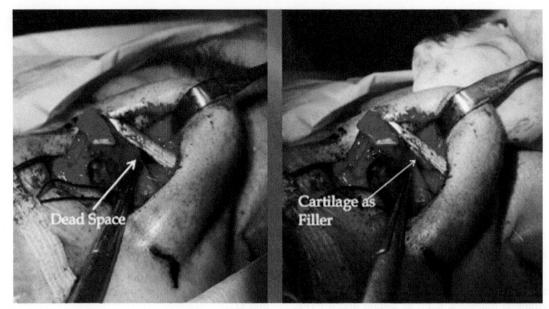

Fig. 19. Sometimes a gap is noted below the implant. The space should be filled up with cartilage to avoid collapse of the implant causing supratip depression.

Alar Flare and Alar Base Plasty: Always Done at the End, if Deemed Necessary

Alar flare and base plasty is always done as the last procedure after the formal rhinoplasty is completed. Usually the flaring improved after structured rhinoplasty is completed (**Fig. 24**). If the flare and/or wide alar base are still present, a simple wedge excision is done (**Fig. 25**). If there is a combination of defect, then correction is a two-dimensional analysis to decrease the flare and narrow the base (**Fig. 26**).

Occasionally a cinching suture using nylon 3-0 is applied as figure-of-eight. Make sure part of

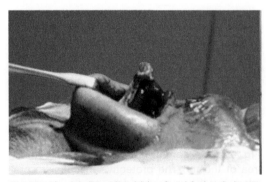

Fig. 20. The implant should be fixed behind the tip grafts. This technique results in the tip and implant complex as one whole unit.

the nasalis muscle is included in the suturing of this maneuver to decrease the tension of the defect. The defect is closed by using nylon 5-0 or 6-0 simple interrupted.[2]

ANCILLARY SOFT TISSUE CONTOURING PROCEDURES
Semi-Lunar Excision of Soft Triangle: For a More Desired Nostril Shape

Some patients have too much fibrofatty tip skin that even with proper structural rhinoplasty the tip still remain bulbous and the shape of the nostril is still unpleasant. The voluminous subtip skin and nostril shape are modified by a semilunar excision of skin and subcutaneous fat (**Fig. 27**). The defect is closed with nylon 6-0 simple interrupted.

Premaxilla Augmentation: Best for Retruded Premaxilla

Most South East Asian noses have small anterior spine hence resulting in retruded premaxilla. Usually after a structural rhinoplasty using a strong SEG, the soft tissue in the premaxilla is displaced anteriorly and superiorly leaving an open space in the premaxilla. The space has to be filled with small cartilage fragments to prevent contracture and retraction of soft tissue resulting in retruded premaxilla. Usually the excess septum and conchal cartilages are used

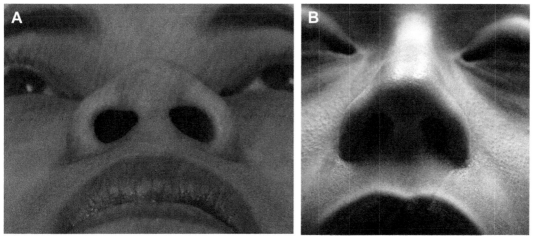

Fig. 21. (*A*) Preoperative monodomal tip. (*B*) One year postoperative. Note the projected bidomal tip already exists.

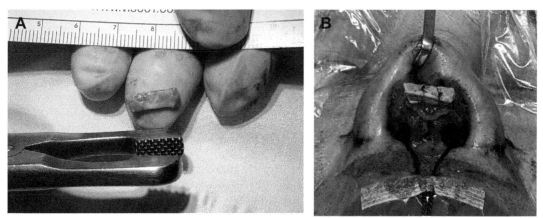

Fig. 22. (*A*) A 10–12 mm × 4–5 mm rectangular tip graft is softened by using cartilage crusher. (*B*) Softened tip graft sutured in place.

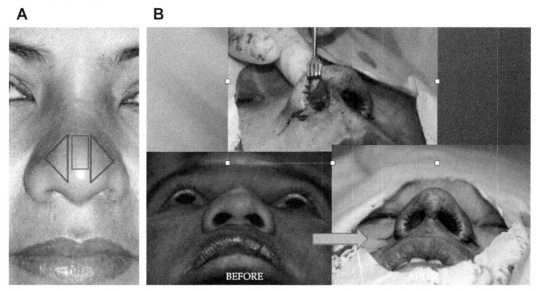

Fig. 23. (*A*) If the tip is still bulbous, the fat surrounding the supratip is trimmed using forceps inserted through the bilateral marginal incision. (*B*) Defatting as the last procedure to contour the tip.

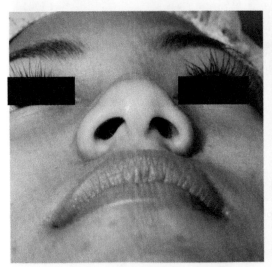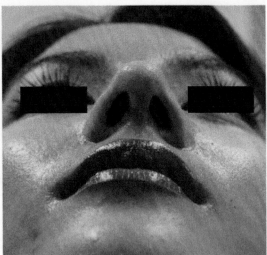

Fig. 24. Usually the flaring of the ala improves after tip projection.

as plump graft. Avoid putting in too much graft because it may give an illusion of rotated tip. Sometimes e-PTFE is used for premaxilla augmentation.

Paranasal Augmentation: Best for Underdeveloped Midface and Deep Nasolabial Fold

There are cases where after completion of rhinoplastic surgery, the midface still appears retruded with deep nasolabial fold. The deep nasolabial fold deformity is easily corrected by augmenting the inferolateral portion of pyriform aperture. Materials range from synthetic (silicon or ePTFE) to autologous cartilage.

A stab incision is done at the gingivobuccal sulcus above the canine root. Blunt dissection is done exposing immediately the periosteum,

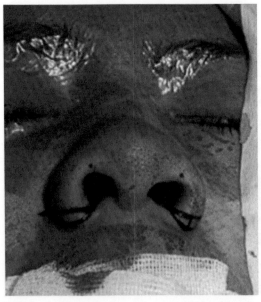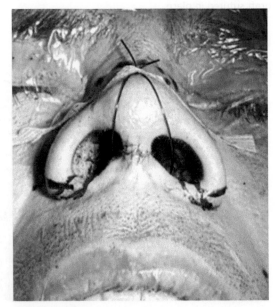

Fig. 25. Markings for the wedge excision in plain alar flare.

Fig. 26. Markings for combination excision for alar flare and wide alar base.

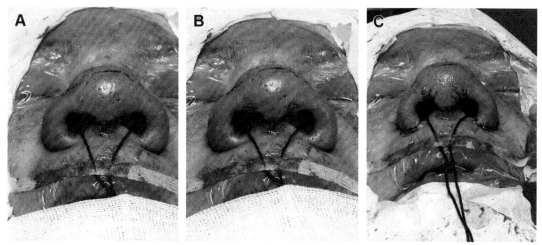

Fig. 27. (*A*) Nostril shape is improved by a semilunar elliptical excision at the soft triangle. (*B*) Markings for excision of skin tissue at the soft triangle preserving the rim skin to prevent notching. (*C*) Closure using nylon 6-0 simple interrupted. Note the immediate change in the nostril shape.

which is elevated snugly to create a cavity lateral to the pyriform aperture. Depending on the mass volume needed a triangular or rectangular shape silicon or e-PTFE is fashioned and inserted snugly into the subperiosteal space. No fixation is required.

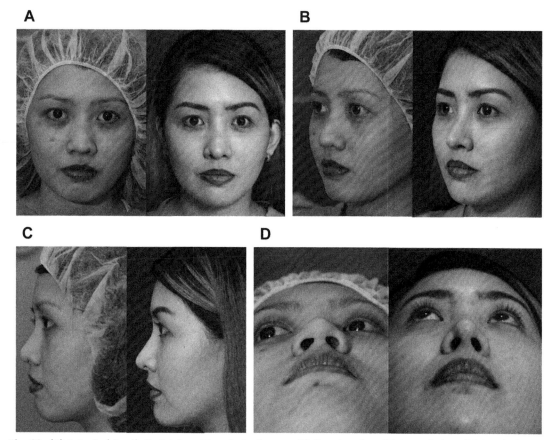

Fig. 28. (*A*) A typical South East Asian rhinoplasty, 5 years. (*B*) Quarter view. (*C*) Lateral view. (*D*) Basal view.

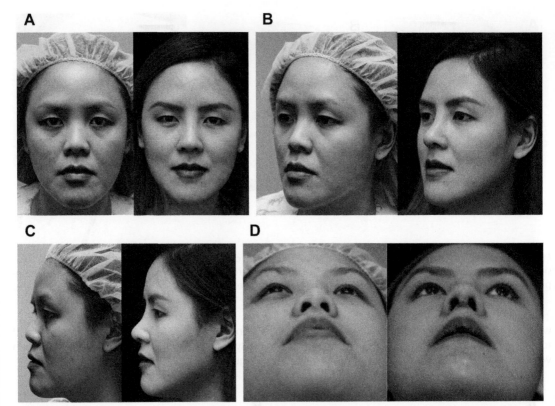

Fig. 29. (*A*) A short and upturned nose 1 week postoperative. (*B*) Oblique view. (*C*) Lateral view. (*D*) Basal view.

SUMMARY

A usual ideal rhinoplasty outcome of a South East Asian nose should be a nose that fits the face with good function and has all the aesthetic landmarks achieved: natural looking dorsum, supratip break, tip, subtip break, columellar show, good alar-columellar relationship, improved premaxilla, improved nostril, and improved alar flare (**Figs. 28** and **29**).

REFERENCES

1. Lee M, Callahan S, Cochran CS. Auricular cartilage: harvest technique and versatility in rhinoplasty. Am J Otolaryngol 2011;32:547–52.

2. Jin HR. Aesthetic plastic surgery of the East Asian face. New York: Thieme; 2016. p. 108–21.

3. Han K, Kim J, Son D, et al. How to harvest the maximal amount of conchal cartilage grafts. J Plast Reconstr Aesthet Surg 2008;61(12):1465–71.

4. Gunter JP, Rohrich RJ, Adams WP. Dallas rhinoplasty, vol. 1. St Louis (MO): QMP; 2007. p. 401–9.

5. Ellenbogen R, Blome DW. Alar rim raising. Plast Reconstr Surg 1992;90(1):28–37.

6. Baladiang DE, Olveda MB, Yap EC. The sail excision technique: a modified alar lift procedure for southeast Asian noses. Philippine Journal Otolaryngol Head Neck Surgery 2010;25:31–7.

7. Yap E. Improving the hanging ala. Facial Plast Surg 2012;28(2):213–7.

8. Byrd HS, Andochick S, Copit S, et al. Septal extension grafts: a method of controlling tip projection shape. Plast Reconstr Surg 1997; 100(4):999–1010.

9. Kim JH, Song JW, Park SW, et al. Effective septal extension graft for Asian rhinoplasty. Arch Plast Surg 2014;41(1):3–11.

10. Porter JP, Tardy ME Jr, Cheng J. The contoured auricular projection graft for nasal tip projection. Arch Facial Plast Surg 1999;1(4):312–5.

11. Kim HS, Park SS, Kim MH, et al. Problems associated with alloplastic materials in rhinoplasty. Yonsei Med J 2014;55(6):1617–23.

Moving?

Make sure your subscription moves with you!

To notify us of your new address, find your **Clinics Account Number** (located on your mailing label above your name), and contact customer service at:

Email: journalscustomerservice-usa@elsevier.com

800-654-2452 (subscribers in the U.S. & Canada)
314-447-8871 (subscribers outside of the U.S. & Canada)

Fax number: 314-447-8029

Elsevier Health Sciences Division
Subscription Customer Service
3251 Riverport Lane
Maryland Heights, MO 63043

Printed and bound by CPI Group (UK) Ltd, Croydon, CR0 4YY

08/05/2025

01864727-0003